The
Principles of

# R U N N I N G

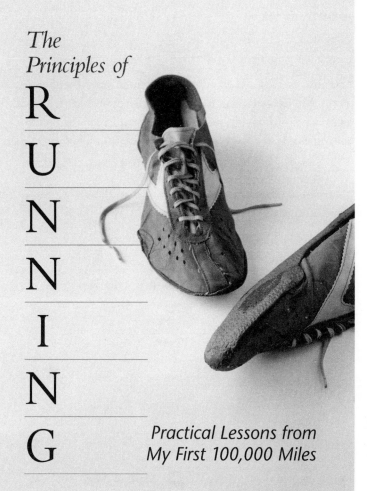

*Practical Lessons from
My First 100,000 Miles*

By Amby Burfoot
Executive Editor, **RUNNER'S** *WORLD.* Magazine
and Winner of the 1968 Boston Marathon

Rodale Press, Inc.
Emmaus, Pennsylvania

Copyright © 1999 by Amby Burfoot
Illustrations copyright © 1999 by Rick Allen

**Cover and Interior Designer:** Joanna Reinhart
**Cover Photographer:** Kurt Wilson

**Library of Congress Cataloging-in-Publication Data**

Burfoot, Amby.
    The principles of running : practical lessons from my first 100,000 miles / by Amby Burfoot.
        p.    cm.
    ISBN 1–57954–038–4 hardcover
    1. Running.    2. Running—Training.    I. Title.
GV1061.B79    1999
796.42—dc21                                                    99–17991

**Distributed to the book trade by St. Martin's Press**

2    4    6    8    10    9    7    5    3    1    hardcover

Visit us on the Web at www.rodalesportsandfitness.com or call us toll-free at (800) 848-4735

─────── Our Purpose ───────

*"We inspire and enable people to improve
their lives and the world around them."*

To Dan and Laura, unfolding miracles who amaze and impress me every day; and to Cristina, who makes it all worthwhile.

# Contents

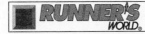

For the latest running news and
training tips, visit our Web site at
www.runnersworld.com

# Introduction

Running is a simple sport, so a simple book ought to be enough to tell you how to do it. This is my attempt to write such a book.

It's called *The Principles of Running* because it doesn't contain everything there is to know about running—only the most important things. Other running experts have written much thicker, more impressive-looking tomes. I couldn't see any reason to duplicate their efforts or to write an even thicker book.

Besides, the runners I've met aren't looking for an encyclopedia. Who has the time? Most runners simply want "the good stuff," as pure and simple as possible. The advice that will guide them to improved performance, better health, fewer injuries, and more enjoyment of running.

I wrote this book because I couldn't locate anything else like it. For years, I've searched for a simple, attractive book I could give to friends, family, and associates to interest them in running. A book that wouldn't intimidate them, a book that was positive and encouraging, a book that was packed full of useful information. I couldn't find anything that fit the bill.

I hope you'll agree that all the most important information is here, and that it's all easy to find. After a quick glance at the table of contents, you should be able to turn to whatever you're looking for.

The information has come from my 35 years of running and the more than 100,000 miles I've covered during that time. In other words, these principles are all road-tested. I've also included the tips, secrets, and strategies I've picked up in 20 years of talking to *Runner's World* readers, from Olympic champions to back-of-the-packers.

During this time, I've learned, for example, that while there are thousands of different kinds of workouts, you need to concentrate on just three or four. You'll find these in part six, Training. Losing weight seems complicated until you understand your metabolism, which is explained in part seven, Weight Loss.

But enough about me and the book itself. How about you? If you're reading these words, you're thinking about beginning to run. Or you've been running for a few years, and now you want to get more involved. You could be a former runner returning to the sport, or a veteran looking for the latest and most scientific training principles.

You could be a high schooler, a woman, or a senior citizen hoping to stay fit and healthy for many years to come. In any and all of these cases, I think you'll find this to be a valuable book. It will instruct you, it will motivate you, it might even inspire you.

Because when you get down to it, it's the big picture that's most important. Don't sweat the small stuff. Get the principles right, and everything else will fall into place.

# ❖ Principles ❖

1. Running is a simple sport and needs only a simple book to tell you how to do things right. This book has been written and organized so that you can easily find the information you need, whether you're a beginning runner or an experienced marathoner.
2. Read this book one chapter at a time, in no particular order. Feel free to skip around. Return to certain chapters to review key points, and save other chapters for another time.
3. Go ahead and "cheat" if you want. Read only the "Principles" section in each chapter to glean the most important advice. No harm done. But you'll gain more background and a greater appreciation for the topic if you read the short chapter material.
4. This book is crammed with tips and suggestions, but don't try to do everything at once. Slow but steady wins the race. Work on just one or two principles at a time.
5. You won't and can't succeed at everything. No one does. Don't get discouraged. Focus your energy on what works for you, and always maintain a positive attitude.

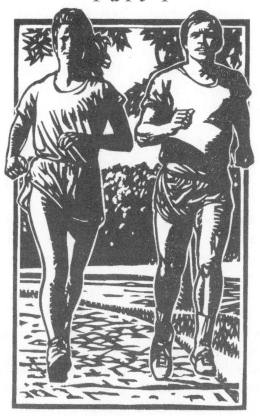

# Part I

# The Joy of Running

# For the Health of It

Decades of medical and scientific research have now proven beyond any doubt that running is one of the healthiest, if not *the* healthiest, exercise. Here are some of the major reasons why.

The simplest and most basic: Running burns more calories in less time than any other exercise. And calorie burning is directly related to oxygen consumption and weight loss, the two most critical aspects of health and fitness. The more oxygen you burn, the more efficient your body's cardiovascular system becomes. And an efficient cardiovascular system resists heart and artery disease.

Weight control is also central to the health goals of many runners, and for good reason. Excess weight is linked with all of the major lifestyle diseases, including heart disease, high blood pressure, and diabetes. And in recent decades, as our lives have gotten ever easier, more sedentary and more computer-driven, the incidence of overweight has climbed alarmingly.

The situation has gotten so bad, in fact, that health officials have declared overweight a national epidemic. They've also figured out why so many people are gaining so much weight, and it's not from eating too much. It's from exercising too little.

To fight this trend (and that unsightly bulge around the middle), you need only become a regular runner. Running is the king of the calorie burners, and you don't need to be fast or graceful. No matter what your pace, you burn roughly 120 calories per mile of running. Run three miles three or four times a week, and you're well on your way to a consistent reduction in weight. Millions of people have done it—including Oprah Winfrey—and you can, too.

The beauty of it is, the program gets easier as you go along. Yes, the first steps and miles can be tough. But once you lose a pound or two, you'll find the running easier, which means you can go farther, which means you'll lose more weight, which means the running gets easier again, so you can go farther again, and lose more weight, which makes the running easier and . . . you get the point.

All you have to do is get started on the program, stick with it for several weeks, and wait for things to get easier. They will. They have to. This isn't some voodoo herbal weight-loss product. These are scientific principles at work, and your body can't disobey them. Like the apple that has to fall *down* from a tree, your body has to lose weight if you're consistently burning more calories than you're consuming.

In addition to these health benefits from running, you'll also feel better. And remarkably, you'll find that you have more energy, not less, every day. That's the beauty of running. You burn calories, lose weight, feel better, and have more energy.

How can you resist giving it a try?

# ❖ Principles ❖

1. Thousands of medical studies over the last five decades have shown that regular exercise can not only extend your life but also make you healthier and more vigorous every day of your life.
2. Running is the simplest, most effective of the regular, lifelong exercise activities. The prime reason: It burns more calories in less time than any other continuous exercise.
3. A regular running program reduces the incidence of the major lifestyle diseases such as heart disease, high blood pressure, and diabetes. It also has a positive influence on many other important health indicators.
4. Humans have been nomadic hunter-gatherers for 99 percent of our existence as a species. Today, we're paying an increasing price for ignoring our ancestry (and our genes) and not moving around as much.
5. Running, which burns roughly 120 calories per mile regardless of your speed, is particularly effective at producing weight loss or helping in a healthy weight-maintenance program.

# The Real Runner's High

Many if not most runners take up running to deal with a physical problem. Losing weight, for example. Who hasn't thought that it would be nice to take off 5 to 10 pounds? Or maybe you have a history of high blood pressure or heart disease.

Good reasons to begin running. But strangely enough, these reasons often fade after several months of regular running. At first, running takes so much effort and willpower that you can't think about anything but the daily struggle. With time, however, a light gradually goes on in your head.

You realize that you feel better when you run. During the run. Immediately after. And throughout the day. You start looking forward to the next day's run because you want that good feeling to flow over you again.

I call this psychological phenomenon runner's high, even though the word is used differently by others. The original runner's high coined 25 years ago was a quasi-mystical, quasi-drugged state. It might have had something to do with opiate-like substances released in the brain after a certain amount and intensity of running. At any rate, few runners actually experienced it, and I doubt you will either.

The runner's high I'm talking about, however, is universal. Every runner knows about it, feels it, and relishes it. It's the feeling you have immediately after a workout: loose, relaxed, refreshed, energized, even exhilarated. And it goes on for hours.

The effect is far from trivial. Studies have shown that runners suffer less from depression than nonrunners, and depression is a major health concern in an overautomated, computer-dominated world that leads many to feel that they have little control over their lives. Running at least gives us some time when we control something—in fact, something important—our bodies.

Regular exercise also gives you a positive, "can do" attitude.

Thousands of runners have attempted a marathon simply because they knew that Oprah Winfrey and Al Gore had finished one. Otherwise, they would never have believed it possible.

And after finishing their own marathons, these people often experience a "Eureka!" moment. "If I can run a marathon," they tell themselves, "then I can dare to start that business I've been thinking about." Or go back to school for a graduate degree.

The daily run also adds clarity to your thinking and often turns into a unique problem-solving time. When you're running, your mind is liberated to roam far and wide. You can develop insights and solutions that would have never occurred to you otherwise.

## ❖ Principles ❖

1. The psychological-emotional benefits of running often turn out to be more compelling and rewarding than the physical benefits. We all need a certain amount of stress-free time during the day, and running provides the perfect escape.
2. Everyone experiences a runner's high during, and especially, after a workout. This high isn't a mystical or drugged state. It's simply the relaxation and revitalization that naturally follows a steady, rhythmic, aerobic workout.
3. Regular running reduces the incidence of depression, a growing problem in the United States. Running may do this through the release of certain neurotransmitters in the brain or simply by giving people more control over their lives.
4. Running seems to improve problem-solving abilities. Many hardworking individuals, from musicians to business people, use their daily runs to concentrate on major roadblocks in their personal, professional, or artistic lives.
5. Running also stimulates creative thinking. This occurs not when you're concentrating on a particular challenge but when a completely unexpected thought pops into your head while you're running. Many runners have had this experience.

# Part II

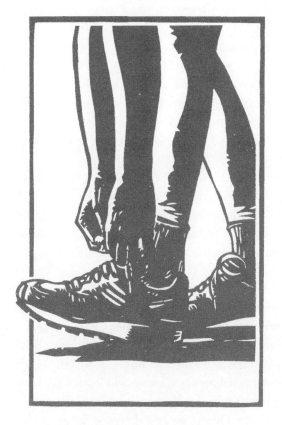

# First Steps

# Getting Started

The most important thing you need to know about running is the least well-known and least discussed: Running is a mental activity, not a physical activity.

If you engage your mind, the body has no choice but to follow along and do what you ask. This means that if you can get on a training program—and stick with it—the body will get in shape.

Too many people have refused to begin running or have quickly dropped out of running programs because they "have no talent for it." Ridiculous. Talent has nothing to do with it. The only thing that matters is mental discipline. Set a goal and a program for yourself, and everything else will follow. Guaranteed. Don't worry about whether you're good enough or fast enough, or whether you're too heavy or too out-of-shape. These things are trifles. They may bother you today, but stick with a running program for several months, and you'll soon forget them.

I always tell beginning runners: Train your brain first. It's much more important than your heart or legs. Once you have your brain signed onto the program, there's only one other thing you have to do: Repeat the story of "The Tortoise and the Hare" to yourself everyday. Concentrate on the moral: Slow but steady wins the race. What worked for the tortoise will work for you, too.

The biggest mistake most beginning runners make is to run too far, too fast. They're afraid others will laugh at them for running too slowly. They want to impress themselves and their friends with their progress. This doesn't work, so forget about it.

Instead, tell yourself to start slowly, then taper off. It's impossible to run too slowly. It's very possible to run too fast . . . and get injured, discouraged, and frustrated. So do the smart thing. Run as slowly as you can. Then slow down a little more.

All beginning running programs are built on a foundation of walking and running. You already know how to walk. The goal is to gradually switch to a little running, then a little more, until you can run steadily for 20 minutes. Repeat this routine three or four times a week, and you're doing the precise amount of exercise recommended by most of the world's medical experts.

At this point, if you choose, you're also ready to do more. You don't have to. But beyond 20 minutes—beyond the basic fitness level—is where you'll find the most exciting and motivating challenges that running has to offer.

Here's how to get to the 20-minute point. You can vary this program almost infinitely, and it's always okay to walk more when you need to. Just remember the slow-but-steady tortoise.

# ❖ Principles ❖

1. Walk 90 seconds, run 30 seconds. Repeat nine more times for a total of 20 minutes. Do four times a week until you're totally comfortable with the workout.
2. Walk 1 minute, run 1 minute. Repeat nine more times for a total of 20 minutes. Do four times a week until totally comfortable.
3. Walk 1 minute, run 2 minutes. Repeat six more times for a total of 21 minutes. Do four times a week until totally comfortable.
4. Walk 1 minute, run 3 minutes. Repeat four more times for a total of 20 minutes. Do four times a week until totally comfortable.
5. Walk 1 minute, run 4 minutes. Repeat three more times for a total of 20 minutes.
6. Walk 1 minute, run 6 minutes. Repeat two more times for a total of 21 minutes.
7. Walk 1 minute, run 8 minutes. Repeat for a total of 18 minutes.
8. Walk 1 minute, run 10 minutes. Repeat for a total of 22 minutes.
9. Walk 1 minute, run 20 minutes slowly, slowly, slowly. Walk 5 minutes for a cooldown. Build up to the point where you can do this four times a week in complete comfort.

# It's Okay to Go Slow

Running is the ultimate tortoise-and-hare activity because the tortoise wins all of the important races. Oh, sure, the hare might get a gold medal at the Olympics or the Boston Marathon. But it's the tortoises who continue to run for decades and often even for a lifetime. And that amounts to a victory in the most important race of your life.

One reason tortoises succeed is that they find a pace that's right for them, both mentally and physically, and they stick to it. No reason to hurry. The slow runners may take longer to reach the finish line than the Olympians, but they get there even more surely than the hares.

An important point about slow runners: They try just as hard as their faster brethren. Many people mistakenly think that slow runners are slow because they don't care to train more or try harder in races. For the most part, this isn't the case (of course, more training will make anyone faster).

Fast runners are fast largely because they have certain genetic gifts. They have an especially strong heart, a high red-blood-cell count, and particularly, the right muscle fibers. Slow runners are slow because they don't have these same gifts—at least not the same amount of them. What's important, though, isn't what the stopwatch tells us. The most important benefits you get from running—the improved health and fitness—are independent of speed. No matter what your speed, if you run, you get the benefits.

The message here is extraordinarily clear: Don't judge your running by your speed. Judge it by how you feel and what your doctor tells you. (Most of the time you don't need a doctor to tell you that the changes in your body and energy are good and healthy ones; that's apparent every day.)

There's a good explanation for this. Even though you may run relatively slowly, your body works at about the same degree of effort as the champions, thereby producing the same physiological changes. That is, when you run a 10-K in 50 or 60 minutes, you perform very nearly the same amount of "work" as a race winner who runs that 10-K in around 30 minutes.

You put as much effort into the race, your heart beats as fast, and your blood circulates in the same manner. The only difference is that the race winner has more "efficient" leg muscles than you, so he breaks the tape and you wait in line for the last bagel.

In most ways, you're exactly the same as the hare. It's only the stopwatch that labels you a tortoise. But don't let it get you down. Run with tortoise pride. And remember: In the longest run of all, your life, you're going to be a winner.

## ❖ Principles ❖

1. Take the "talk test." Run at a pace that allows you to conduct a normal conversation with your training partners. No gasping allowed. That's too fast.
2. When measuring pulse rate, keep it in the range of 60 to 70 percent of your maximum pulse rate. This is the aerobic pulse that provides virtually all the workout benefits you need and want. Obtain your maximum pulse rate by subtracting your age from 220.
3. If you don't have a heart-rate monitor, use the Perceived Exertion Scale, and run at an effort level of 5 or 6. The Perceived Exertion Scale goes from 1 to 10, where 1 is a slow walk; 2, a brisk walk; and 10, an all-out race effort. If you rate your effort a 5 or 6, you will be in the moderate aerobic range you want.
4. Don't worry that you're going too slowly. You're not, and you can't run too slowly. All running qualifies as vigorous activity, according to scientific principles, and brings you maximum benefits.
5. Run comfortably and run for a lifetime. This should be your major goal.

# Good Form

Every runner wants to run with perfect form. To look like a gazelle bounding across the endless plains. Or something like that. Anything graceful and flowing. Nothing awkward and clunky.

It's a pretty picture, but forget it. Research shows that it doesn't matter what you look like when you run. While many scientists have searched for decades to uncover the secret of perfect running form, they've just about given up the chase. Some Olympic champions have run like gazelles while others have run like elephants. Either way, their running form didn't have much effect on how fast they could pick up their feet and move them forward.

Turns out about the only things that matter, in terms of pure speed, are your genetics and your biochemistry. And you can't do anything about either. So don't worry about it. Instead, concentrate on good form.

And don't be a slave to the advice you've been hearing for years: Pick up your knees, lengthen your stride, lean forward, pump your arms. These techniques work great for some runners. Until they get beaten by someone with an upright body carriage; short, shuffling strides; and minimal arm movement.

Instead of aiming for a meaningless ideal, you'll do much better to run the way that feels most relaxed, natural, and comfortable to you. Run the way you remember running in your childhood—loose and carefree. Don't look around and compare your running form with anyone else's.

That said, there may be reasons other than speed to evaluate your running form. You might be suffering from frequent injuries, you might have sore neck and shoulder muscles, or you might be developing a knot in your calf muscle.

These and other problems could inhibit your enjoyment of running and, worse, lead to injuries that prevent you from running as regularly and as pain-free as you'd like. Since the ability to run consistently without injuries forms the foundation of all of running's benefits, it makes sense to develop a running form that prevents injuries.

Most running injuries happen as a result of impact shock—the pounding of your feet on the roads. To decrease the pounding, use a shuffle stride rather than bouncing along from one leg to the other. A short stride also reduces pounding, as does running with an erect carriage, which feels comfortable to many runners and prevents pain along the neck, back, and hips.

To introduce yourself to this erect, short-striding form, begin at a slow walk on a road or track. Then increase your walking speed. Increase it again. When you're going so fast that you can no longer walk—when you have to run—maintain the exact same movements you used while walking, but let yourself ease into a run. This low-key, relaxed running form is probably the one that will work best for you.

## ❖ Principles ❖

1. Run tall and erect, with your ears over your shoulders over your hips over your heels.
2. Look straight ahead (okay, just slightly down), not at the road immediately in front of your feet.
3. Keep your shoulders relaxed. Let your arms swing comfortably at your sides.
4. Don't lean forward, don't run on your toes, and don't bounce.
5. Lift your knee just enough to get your leg moving forward. Don't reach out and ahead with your front foot. Let it return naturally to the road right under your knee.
6. Smile. Research has shown that a happy runner is a relaxed, efficient runner, and a smile will make you feel happy. It will also send a good message to everyone who sees you running and will likely make them smile.

# Motivation

Motivation is the name of the game, period. This is one of the primary reasons I've argued that running is as much a mental activity as a physical one. The key to success is keeping yourself motivated. If you succeed at maintaining your motivation, you'll succeed at running and get everything you want from it.

I'm always surprised that we "experts" have dozens, if not hundreds of tips, about training, nutrition, and injury-prevention, but precious little of our wisdom is devoted to motivation. It should be the other way around. Give someone the motivation to run, and he will eventually figure out all the other stuff. Motivation should be at the top of our lists, not the bottom.

You may have a little piece of paper somewhere on which you've written down things like "Lose 10 pounds" or "Run the Hometown 5-K" or "Get in shape to jog three miles with Frank at Thanksgiving."

Great. Now add another goal. Write down "Stay motivated." Without motivation, you'll soon forget why you're running, find excuses to miss workouts, and gradually fall out of your exercise habit.

How do you stay motivated? Start by reminding yourself of the many reasons for running. You'll feel better, look better, be healthier, and have more energy for work and family.

Find a compatible running partner. This is one of the best tricks I know. Don't race each other during workouts; just shoot the breeze for 30, 40, or 60 minutes of comfortable, enjoyable running. Even if you and your friend can only get together once or twice a week, you can both help motivate each other.

In this digital age, there are many electronic means to contact other runners and join "virtual" running communities. At Runner's World Online (www.runnersworld.com), we feature many forums for different interest groups. You can also join Internet listservs, which you can access through your Internet provider, where you will meet hundreds, if not thousands, of other runners like you.

Pull out all the tricks you can think of. Collect inspirational quotes and put them on your refrigerator or in your office. Seek out stories of other runners and individuals who have overcome significant obstacles to succeed at their quests. Set lots of attainable short-term goals. Make them easy, so you'll be sure to achieve them. When you achieve one, quickly establish your next one.

Don't set unrealistic performance goals like "Run a mile in seven minutes." Instead, aim to "Run 15 miles this week." It takes only motivation and discipline to run a certain amount every week.

When you do succeed, reward yourself with a pat on the back or something more materialistic—a new running shirt, a meal at a nice restaurant, a book or a video, a trip to a special race or event. Remember: Maintaining your motivation is crucial to your success, and rewards are very motivating. In short, be good to yourself.

## ❖ Principles ❖

1. Set realistic goals and reach them. Don't go for records. Aim for results that will bring you maximum satisfaction.
2. Find a compatible running partner to run with once or twice a week. Don't compete with each other. Enjoy the time together and do everything you can to keep each other motivated throughout the week.
3. Enter occasional races to increase your motivation and to feel the excitement that accompanies races. This will have a spillover effect to keep you motivated for weeks afterward. Think about picking one fun, local race and making it "your" race. Run it every year.
4. Read inspirational stories about other runners or other people who have overcome obstacles to achieve success in their given field. If these people can do it, so can you.
5. Seek out new places to run and other new running adventures. Consider trails, relays, mountain races, or marathons.

# Aches and Pains

Every runner gets aches and pains at one time or another. To some degree, you must accept them. They go with the turf . . . and especially the road. Indeed, the repetitive pounding of your legs on hard asphalt or concrete surfaces is often the cause of those temporary aches and pains.

When I say temporary, I mean soreness that fades away after three to four days. That's the normal course of generalized muscle soreness as opposed to genuinely injured muscle tissues. The best way to treat simple muscle soreness is to stop running for several days. If that pretty much clears up your complaint, then you know it was nothing serious to begin with, and it's perfectly okay to return to your training routine.

To help deal with muscle aches, experts recommend RICE—rest, ice, compression, and elevation. In my experience, the first two of these are by far the most useful. I've just mentioned how several days of rest will often cure muscle soreness.

When using ice on an injury, here's the best approach. Try to ice the injured area for 15 minutes at a time, at least three times a day. More often is better, longer isn't, as it can actually damage tissue in your skin. To protect the skin, put a thin cotton towel between the ice and your injury site. Runners often apply ice in one of the following forms: a paper cup that they keep stored in the freezer, peeling back the paper with each use to expose more ice; a bag of frozen corn or frozen peas; or a commercial ice gel that is flexible enough to be contoured to the injury site.

Compression and elevation don't seem very practical for an active runner, but you can certainly use an elastic bandage to compress and support an injured muscle. And perhaps at the end of the day, you can elevate your injury while icing it.

Most over-the-counter sports balms produce little effect. They may warm, and even irritate, the skin, but they have never been shown to do much good within the actual injured muscle tissue. Anti-inflammatories, like aspirin, ibuprofen, and naproxen sodium, can be helpful as long as you use them while you're resting your injury. They won't do you any good—in fact, they could worsen your condition—if you're simply using them to mask the pain and continue running.

Massage, including self-massage, is a great boon to many runners. Again, you shouldn't use it in place of rest and other injury-resolving approaches but in addition to them. In recent years, a number of specific "sticks" and other knobby tools have made their way onto the market to help runners massage themselves more effectively in hard-to-reach areas. Massage unquestionably relaxes muscles and sometimes helps to loosen up knots, adhesions, and other tight spots that cause pain and loss of motion.

## ❖ Principles ❖

1. Occasional muscular aches and pains are an inevitable part of running. Don't let them frustrate you. Learn to cope with them and resolve them.
2. Rest is always the first step. When you have unusual muscle soreness, take several days off from running. Even try to avoid excessive walking on these days. Give your muscles a real break.
3. At the same time, ice the sore muscles several times a day for about 15 minutes. Use an inexpensive flexible gel wrap, an ice pack, or even a small bag of frozen vegetables.
4. Anti-inflammatories can also prove helpful in relieving slight muscle injuries (acetaminophen is a painkiller but not an anti-inflammatory). Take the recommended dosage around the clock for as long as a week, then stop to test your sore muscles.
5. Return very gradually to your running program. Consider a several-mile walk for your first workout. Remember: You have all the time in the world. Get over your aches and pains first, then get back to running.

# Blisters

You can't run without getting the occasional blister. It's simply a recreational hazard—the inevitable result when your feet spend so much time working so hard inside a pair of shoes. You can, however, learn to minimize the number and severity of the blisters you get, and many runners come very close to eliminating them entirely.

Blisters are caused by friction, the rubbing of your skin against another surface, so anything that reduces friction inside your socks or shoes will help fight blisters. Buying shoes that fit properly is the first step. Be sure to try on several pairs, walk or jog around in them, and purchase the pair that feels most comfortable and produces the least rubbing against your feet. Pay particular attention to any seams inside the shoe, as these could cause trouble down the road.

While some runners prefer running without socks, the vast majority use socks, and there are many arguments *for* wearing socks (not the least of which are cleanliness and the fight against shoe and foot odor). In recent years, the fibers used in socks have improved tremendously, and much of the old advice about socks (buy wool or cotton) is no longer true.

Surprisingly, synthetic fibers are now the materials of choice. Look for breathable athletic socks made from 100-percent-polyester fibers. These socks will draw sweat away from your feet, eliminating the moisture that is a major cause of friction and blisters.

Some socks now claim additional blister-prevention features. Socks with two layers, for example, are said to let the layers, rather than your feet, absorb friction. Try them to see if they work for you. One trick of the trade: Wear your socks inside out so that any seams are on the outside, where they can't do much damage.

Since sweat and other moisture increases the threat of blisters (not to mention athlete's foot), it's always a good idea to do whatever you can to keep your feet dry. Many runners find that powdering their feet before running is very effective. Others prefer "slicking" their feet with petroleum jelly and other, similar products to reduce friction. One recent study even found that putting an antiperspirant on your feet reduces the risk of blisters.

If you do develop blisters during a workout or race, you'll want to treat them properly afterward so that you can quickly return to your training routine. Minor blisters that aren't causing a lot of irritation should be left alone to heal. The skin over the blister is as good a protective covering as you'll find.

Blisters that contain a large pool of fluid should be drained and bandaged. You can do this yourself. Find a sewing needle, wash your hands, and wipe the needle with alcohol to sterilize it. Then carefully puncture the blister at one edge and gently force the fluid out with your fingers. When finished, bandage the blister to keep it clean and protect against infection.

## ❖ Principles ❖

1. You can't run regularly without getting occasional blisters, but you can learn to keep them to a minimum. With proper care, blisters should never interfere with your running.
2. Selecting the right pair of shoes is a crucial first step. Try on several pairs, walk or jog in them, and buy the pair that feels the most comfortable and produces the least amount of rubbing against your feet. Be sure to check that the shoes have no inseams that could cause problems.
3. Socks are another important preventive. Buy breathable athletic socks made of 100-percent-polyester fibers such as Coolmax.
4. Dry feet are generally healthy, blister-free feet, so many runners powder their feet before running to prevent both athlete's foot and blisters. Alternatives: using petroleum jelly or similar products to reduce friction inside the shoe.
5. If you do develop blisters, leave small ones alone. Larger blisters should be punctured and drained with a sterilized needle and bandaged to ensure cleanliness and protection against infection.

# The 10-Percent Rule

The 10-percent rule (10PR) is one of the most important and time-proven principles in running. It states that you should never increase your weekly mileage by more than 10 percent over the previous week.

The 10PR gains its importance from the fact that the vast majority of running injuries are overuse injuries. They occur when you run too much or increase your weekly training program too quickly. Say you've been running 15 miles a week. For some reason—perhaps you want to prepare for an upcoming race or you just feel that you're ready—you decide to pick up your training. Instead of running 5 miles three times a week, you manage to fit in five 5-milers. Your training increases from 15 miles a week to 25 miles a week—a 67 percent increase.

The week of the race, your knee starts throbbing. By Saturday, you're hobbling. You can't ignore the handwriting on the wall. You're not going to be able to run the Sunday morning race. You have a knee injury.

For runners, the biggest enemy is often their own energy and enthusiasm. You're feeling great, so you figure that you can handle more training. A friend has challenged you to enter a race. Everyone in your department at work has decided to get in shape for an upcoming charity run. Or maybe you've been bitten by the marathon bug.

Events like these are big motivators, so you plunge excitedly into the training. Great—except for one thing. Your body doesn't share in your enthusiasm. It follows one simple, unchanging principle: gradual adaptation to stress.

The gradual adaptation principle is one of the many examples of the body's genius. Without it, no one could ever climb Mount Everest, swim the English Channel, or run a marathon. With it there are almost no limits to what you can achieve. But you can't bend the rules, or the system breaks, and you get an injury or pick up a cold or suddenly become fatigued.

Follow the 10PR, on the other hand, and your body gets stronger and fitter. If you're running 10 miles a week now, and you want to increase your training, run 11 miles next week. And 12 the week after that. And 13 the week after that. This may look like agonizingly slow progress, but in just 8 to 10 weeks, you could be running 20 miles a week.

Continue on the same path, and you'll be running 40 miles a week just four months after you started building up from 10. And 40 miles a week, believe me, is a lot of running. It can take you anywhere you want to go.

Once again, the race goes to the tortoise. In running, you will almost always win if you follow the path of slow-but-sure.

# ❖ Principles ❖

1. Increase your weekly training mileage by no more than 10 percent per week. For example, run 20 miles one week, 22 the next, 24 the next, and so on.
2. When increasing mileage, add to the distance of your current runs rather than adding more days of running. This method will continue to give you the rest and recovery days you need.
3. Don't increase mileage and speed at the same time. When increasing mileage, keep running at your current pace. When increasing speed, you should actually decrease weekly mileage.
4. Also follow the 10-percent rule when building up the length of your long runs. Don't, for example, jump from 8 miles to 12 miles. Take it more gradually.
5. Consider running by time rather than mileage. This makes it much easier to follow the 10-percent rule. If you do 120 minutes of training one week, you can do 132 the next. If your long run is 50 minutes one week, you can increase it to 55 minutes the following week.

# Running and Walking

A few years ago, many runners regarded walking as a morally bankrupt, poor cousin to running. You only walked if you were lazy and undisciplined. Anyone with real determination ran. Fortunately, attitudes have changed as many runners have learned how running and walking can be combined into a healthful program.

To my way of thinking, there's only one thing wrong with walking: Often it isn't "vigorous" enough—the word scientists use to describe exercise that's guaranteed to produce beneficial results. Well, there is another thing. Walking takes too long.

When you combine running and walking, however, you have the perfect exercise program. Here's why: The running makes your workouts vigorous and time-efficient; the walking allows you to go farther. The whole is greater than the sum of the parts.

Not only that, but when you look closely, you realize that mixing walking and running is part of virtually all running programs. The beginning runner alternates several minutes of walking with one minute of running to gradually improve his condition. The Olympic runner alternates very fast, short runs with slow jogs or walks (interval training). This training has long been accepted as the best way to achieve world-class results. And the ultra-runner—those adventurers who don't think 26 miles is far enough—mix running and walking to help them cover 50, 100, sometimes even 1,000 miles.

I've found from personal experience that the run-walk system is also perfect for those times when I'm recovering from a slight injury or when I'm tired and need an easy day of training. On these days, I might run 4 minutes, walk 1 minute, and then repeat until I've finished a 30- to 60-minute workout. Piece of cake.

When I'm training for a marathon, I often follow a nine-to-one plan: nine minutes of running, followed by one minute of walking. The short periods of walking provide a wonderful break in what can otherwise be a tedious and difficult workout. This program is now the best one I know for first-time marathoners trying to figure out how they can train themselves to keep going for the full 26.2 miles.

Olympic marathoner Jeff Galloway has pioneered a similar system that works miracles during a marathon. He has trained runners to run from mile mark to mile mark, and then to take a 60-second walking break while they drink fluids or chew energy bars. Galloway's system has taken many who never imagined they could complete the distance and turned them into marathoners.

Galloway's program highlights the power of the run-walk regimen. If it works during a marathon, it will work for almost any training run. It can help you cover more miles, but it can also help you run stronger and faster.

In other words, you can tailor run-walk training to do exactly what you want it to do. And that's a great reason to give it a try.

# ❖ Principles ❖

1. Walk 90 seconds, run 30 seconds. Repeat nine more times for a total of 20 minutes. Do this four times a week until you're totally comfortable with the workout. This is a great way to get started on a beginning runner's program.
2. Run for 4 minutes, then walk for 1 minute. Repeat 11 more times. This is a great way to do a steady 60-minute workout.
3. Run slowly for one minute, run medium-fast for two minutes, run slowly for one minute, then walk for one minute. Repeat 8 to 12 times. This is a great way to do a modified tempo-training workout that will improve your 10-K and half-marathon times.
4. Run slowly for one minute, run fast for one minute, run slowly for two minutes, then walk for one minute. Repeat 8 to 12 times. This is a great speed workout to improve your 5-K times.
5. Run slowly for nine minutes, walk for one minute. Repeat 9 to 18 times, gradually increasing the distance you cover. This is a great way to do a long run as you prepare for a marathon.

Part III

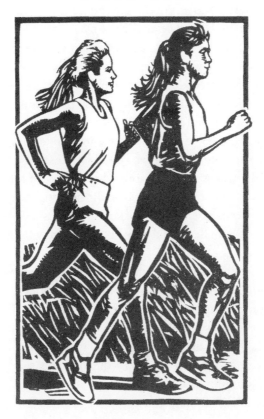

Women

# Safety

As athletes who enjoy the great outdoors, runners must be ever wary of the threats out there—everything from cars and trucks to grizzly bears. These exist in varying degrees, depending on where you live and run, and it would be stupid not to acknowledge that exercising near them can be dangerous. Fortunately, it takes only a few commonsense precautions to greatly minimize the risks and dangers.

Women, of course, face another threat: men. I would prefer not to have to write this chapter. I would prefer that women could run in all the places and situations where men can run and never have to give a passing thought to their personal safety. I would prefer that women, who have broken so many shackles in recent decades, could run freely and fully liberated at any time and in any place they choose.

But they can't. And it would be stupid for any woman not to acknowledge the precautions she must take. Forewarned is forearmed. Run safe, not sorry.

Whenever possible, a woman runner should run with someone else. A small group that includes several male runners is the ideal, but simply running with one other woman is a big step in the right direction. Running with a dog is another option. The goal, obviously, is to avoid running alone.

If you can't find a running partner, run during daylight in the safest place you can find, one with lots of other runners, cyclists, or walkers. Don't run alone in isolated areas, no matter how much the forests and trails might beckon. Don't wear headphones and don't run in the dark. Think about buying a treadmill or joining a club where you can use its treadmills.

Consider carrying a self-defense spray. Sprays with pepper gas are small, easy to carry, and very effective at causing pain and temporary blindness without permanent damage. Test your spray in the backyard to make sure you know how it works. Whenever you go out on a run that makes you feel even slightly uneasy, clip the spray to the waistband of your running shorts.

Try to look strong and confident while you're running. If someone approaches, don't look away. Look at the person briefly to size him up, let your eyes wander around a little, then look again to let him know that you're serious about his presence. Don't look down and appear timid; try to look self-assured.

If you're attacked, your legs are your best weapon—they are much stronger than your upper body, especially since you're a runner. If you're pushed down, roll onto your back, not your stomach, and kick as furiously as you can. At the same time, scream and yell for help. This will frighten your assailant and hopefully bring you quick assistance.

# ❖ Principles ❖

1. The outdoor world is full of risks, most of which can be mini-mized by following simple, commonsense strategies. Women, however, must also be on the alert for attacks by men. They happen infrequently, but they're a genuine threat.
2. Whenever possible, run with someone else, particularly with a group that includes at least one man. Running with another woman friend is also far better than running alone. As an alter-native, run with a dog.
3. If you can't find anyone to accompany you, run during daylight in a place with lots of other people. There's strength in numbers.
4. Never wear headphones. Never run in the dark. Don't run in areas you don't know well. Don't run alone on trails and other remote places. Carry pepper spray, and don't let yourself get forced into someone's car.
5. If you are attacked and pushed to the ground, roll on your back and use your strong runner's legs to kick furiously. Kick and scream, kick and scream.

# Menstruation

A woman runner is naturally curious about how her menstrual period and running will affect each other. She might wonder if running will make the menstrual flow heavier and cramps worse. And if she runs a race during her period, will it affect her performance?

Physicians agree that a normal menstrual period should never force a woman to skip her workouts. In fact, exercise may reduce some of the pain and bloating associated with your periods. And most women runners find that a moderate run lessens the cramps experienced by 60 to 75 percent of all women.

Contrary to what many women may think, there are no real differences in performance due to the stage of the menstrual cycle. Some women experience an increased shortness of breath the week before their periods, which corresponds to the week after ovulation. This comes from elevated levels of the hormone progesterone.

Common sense and nutritional guidelines indicate that women runners should pay special attention to their intake of iron and calcium. The iron will prevent anemia; the calcium will guarantee strong bone growth.

Most of the research about women, sports, and menstrual periods has focused on a condition that has come to be known as the female athlete triad. The triad refers to the connection between training (and other stresses), diet, and amenorrhea—the complete absence of menstrual periods. Amenorrhea is a concern because it can lead to osteoporosis, a major women's health issue.

The women most susceptible to the triad seem to be runners, gymnasts, and dancers because all three activities reward women for thinness. In running, a lean body correlates with a high aerobic capacity and fast running.

Amenorrhea is far different than irregular periods. Irregular periods are common for many women, and women runners tend to have more irregular periods than their nonexercising counterparts.

Irregular periods alone don't signal that anything is wrong. They may simply represent a natural response to your training.

Amenorrhea, on the other hand, indicates that something has gone wrong and that you might not be depositing new calcium to your bones as you should be. Any woman who has no periods for a prolonged time should consult with her physician.

It is important to note that some women assume that if they are amenorrheic, they cannot get pregnant. This is true most of the time, but not all of the time. If you are not interested in conceiving, you should use your normal method of birth control.

Fortunately, a simple treatment plan often puts an end to amenorrhea. A woman runner who decreases her training intensity and increases her caloric intake generally returns to regular periods quite quickly. Her physician will probably also recommend the use of calcium supplements just to be on the safe side and may even recommend hormone replacement therapy.

# ❖ Principles ❖

1. It's okay to run during your menstrual period. In fact, many women runners find that it helps keep them emotionally balanced and steady while reducing menstrual cramps.
2. Women runners are more likely to have irregular periods than sedentary women, but this alone doesn't signal that anything is wrong. Menstrual periods differ widely among all women.
3. A complete lack of menstrual periods, called amenorrhea, represents a health risk and should be treated. It tends to strike hard-training runners who also restrict their diets. Amenorrhea does not prevent pregnancy.
4. Generally, periods for amenorrheic women will return after a reduction in running intensity and an increase in caloric intake.
5. It's always a good idea for women runners to pay special attention to their intake of iron and calcium. The iron will prevent anemia; the calcium will help to ensure healthy bone growth.

# Pregnancy

Thirty years ago, the sight of a pregnant woman jogging would have sent people to their telephones for frantic calls to the police demanding that the crazy lady be protected from herself. Today, expectant mothers are encouraged to continue their fitness programs with just a few precautions.

And why not? The aerobically inclined mother-to-be is still, in all likelihood, burning far fewer calories than her ancestral counterpart. The cavemom had to trot over the African veldt for most of the day to keep up with her nomadic tribe.

In other words, evolutionary biology has had plenty of time to prepare women for the twin rigors of child-carrying and exercising. And, needless to say, biology has thought of all of the contingencies and prepared thoroughly.

Many women, and especially their family members, nonetheless worry endlessly about the imagined risks of running while pregnant. What about miscarriage? What about heat and dehydration? And how is the fetus going to get enough oxygen if you're forcing so much of it to your leg muscles?

A recent study of nearly 3,000 women who had just given birth found, however, that the mothers' levels of exercise didn't cause more birth problems or lower birth weights among the newborns. Even the mothers who exercised heavily and worked long hours delivered healthy babies if they followed other appropriate guidelines.

Miscarriage is a threat primarily during the first trimester of pregnancy. Research has never shown any connection between exercise and miscarriage, but you should certainly get off your feet anytime you experience unexpected cramps or bleeding. And, of course, see your physician immediately for a checkup.

Some worry that all of the running around will bounce the fetus too much, causing it physical harm. This is not a problem, as the fetus is perfectly protected in the uterus.

Similarly, your baby will get plenty of blood and oxygen while you exercise. Your body has been designed to ensure that this happens. You'll get tired and be forced to stop exercising long before your baby suffers any loss.

Naturally, you'll want to watch your nutrition during pregnancy. It's especially important to drink plenty of fluids, including milk, and to eat dairy products and lots of carbohydrates.

Some doctors advise against running fast or running long, particularly in hot weather. While these are more theoretical than real concerns, it only makes sense to follow them. Don't expect to set personal records or finish multiple marathons while pregnant.

After giving birth, you should once again rely on common sense in deciding when to return to running. Don't force yourself back too soon, and be sure to follow a slow, gradual comeback. In a few months, with the help of a jogging stroller, you and your new training partner can enjoy the great outdoors together.

# ❖ Principles ❖

1. Running is a simple, natural act, and pregnancy is a complex but wholly natural condition. Millions of years of evolution have guaranteed that the two are completely compatible.
2. When pregnant, it makes sense to run shorter distances with less intensity. This isn't the time to try for new records or to enter a lot of marathons.
3. Listen to your body at all times. When you feel good, exercise a little longer. When you feel tired, do less. If you have any cramps or bleeding, see your doctor at once.
4. Pregnancy demands that you stay hydrated, consume as many dairy products as you can, and maintain a high-carbohydrate diet with ample calories.
5. After delivery, wait two weeks to two months before running again. Don't push it. Follow a slow, gradual comeback program.

# Menopause

With the running boom still gaining strength and millions of baby-boom women suddenly finding themselves at home with an "empty nest," more fifty-something women are running than ever before. And no matter whether these women are experienced runners or beginners just covering their first tentative miles, they all have to deal at some point with the effects of menopause.

For many, it's a troubling experience. What good can you say about losing energy, gaining weight, living with hot flashes, and feeling that your body is no longer under your control? At the same time, most women and most experts agree that staying fit at menopause may be the single best thing you can do to maintain your physical and emotional health.

But it does take an attitude adjustment. You can't expect to run as fast as you did when you were younger. And since runners gauge themselves (too harshly, most of the time) by their running pace, this can be a depressing reality. So remember, even if you're slower than you were 20 years ago, you're still faster than 99.9 percent of this planet's women of your age.

And what's the point of time comparisons anyway? A main reason for running is to be as fit and healthy as you can be at any age. Don't compare yourself with others. Don't even compare yourself with the former you. Simply do the most and the best you can with where you are now.

Fifty-something women who are thinking about starting a running program will find dozens of reasons why they shouldn't and can't. They'll have every excuse in the book, from "I'm too busy" to "How can I run when I have to deal with menopause and all the strange changes in my body?"

Here's the answer: There's no better time than today. Paradoxically, those times when you're feeling the worst are often the best times to turn the corner and move toward positive change.

Excuses are easy to find and comforting, but only action can make your life better.

Women runners at menopause should, of course, consult with their doctors and pursue every medical option appropriate to them. While not right for everyone, hormone replacement therapy can protect you from heart disease, bone loss, and colon cancer.

A strength-training program can also do much for a body that seems to be getting weaker in so many ways. Strength training is a perfect complement to the aerobic fitness you'll get from running.

Any way you look at it, the decision really isn't that difficult. Either you choose to stay fit no matter what changes are going on in your body, or you choose not to exercise and become a pawn of your body's biology, with no answering voice of your own.

# ❖ Principles ❖

1. Every woman experiences menopause differently, but there's almost never a good reason to give up running. Nor are there enough good excuses to prevent you from starting to run.
2. You may need to adjust your thinking. Don't compare yourself with others or even with your younger self. Don't worry about time, pace, and performance. Run for yourself. Only yourself. And do it today.
3. Consider a modest strength-training program to complement your running. The two work wonderfully together, especially during menopause.
4. Consult with your primary-care physician to explore medical options that might be appropriate for you. Hormone therapy can offer some protection against heart disease and bone loss.
5. Don't let age or biology prevent you from living a full, active, healthy life. You're never too old to benefit from a regular exercise program. The alternative—simply letting your body slide down a long, depressing slope—is really no alternative at all. Don't let life pass you by.

# Special Concerns

One reason why so many women have taken up running and succeeded so spectacularly is that running presents few obstacles. You don't have to weigh 250 pounds, stand seven feet tall, or swing a bat like Mark McGwire. You do need determination, discipline, and good planning skills—qualities that women have in spades.

Still, women do have size, strength, and hormonal differences from men, and these can affect your running. Here's what you need to know about them.

**Shoes.** Women have smaller, narrower feet than men. Even if you find a men's shoe that fits you lengthwise, it might still be too wide for you, especially in the heel. Heel slippage is something you definitely want to avoid.

So the first step is to try on shoes that are made for women. If nothing feels right, by all means try on men's shoes as well. Every foot is different, and you might feel more comfortable in a men's shoe. Be sure that the shoe has enough flexibility for you. Because women are smaller and lighter than men, some men's shoes don't flex easily when women run in them.

**Apparel.** Women have had a dramatic impact on the running apparel market. For a time, one or two women-owned companies were the only ones making running clothes tailored specifically to a woman's body. Now everyone is. Whether you want tight, aerodynamic clothing or a looser, fuller look, you should be able to find a fit and cut that feels right to you.

**Sports bras.** Experts recommend that women runners wear sports bras when they work out. Wearing a sports bra will make you feel more comfortable. Make sure your bra has no inseams or metal clips that could chafe you. When trying on a sports bra in the store, jump up and down to see if it does what it's supposed to do. Women with small breasts often prefer compression bras, while large-breasted women feel better in bras that encapsulate each breast.

**Wider hips.** Women have wider hips than men, which gives them more angularity from the hips to the knees. Some physiologists have speculated that this makes women more prone to knee injuries than men, though no research studies have ever proved this. Nonetheless, it makes a lot of sense for women runners to do quadriceps-strengthening exercises.

**Eating disorders.** Women suffer much more than men from anorexia nervosa and bulimia, the two most common eating disorders. Physicians once viewed these as strictly nutritional problems but now realize they are often related to social pressures and psychological issues. Women runners with an eating disorder need plenty of emotional support from their families and possibly professional help. You can help them, or yourself, with assurances that a well-balanced diet is essential to long-term health and athletic success.

# ❖ Principles ❖

1. Women are lighter than men and have narrower feet, so they should pay particular attention to buying shoes that fit properly.
2. Women should run in sports bras that don't chafe. The bras don't prevent sagging breasts (which aren't caused by running anyway) but they will make you feel more comfortable.
3. Because women have wider hips and a bigger "Q angle" (from the hips to the knees), they should do quadriceps-strengthening exercises to help stabilize the knees and keep them injury-free.
4. Women must realize that eating disorders pose a threat to their long-term health and athletic success. Only a complete, well-balanced diet can contribute the calories and nutrients that an active woman needs on a daily basis.
5. Women are much more like men than different from them, which is why so many women runners have succeeded brilliantly in the sport. What works for men—training, nutrition, injury prevention—will also work for women.

# Part IV

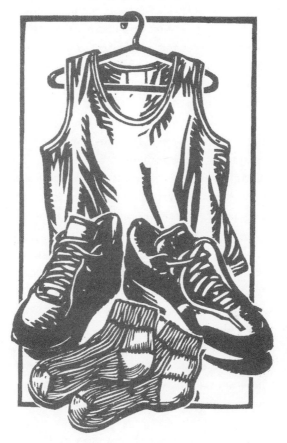

Equipment

# Shoes

Runners have it good. Our sport requires almost no special equipment, and the gear you do need is relatively inexpensive. The one essential ingredient, of course, is good shoes.

The right pair of shoes won't just look good, feel good, and help you run in comfort. They will also help you prevent injuries. This is why it's so important that you find the right pair.

The most important step in buying the right shoes is finding the pair that fits you the best. The most advanced, most feature-laden shoes in the world won't work well if they don't fit your feet. Finding the right pair takes time and effort—you may even have to visit several stores—but it's well worth the investment. A good pair of shoes will last six to eight months (approximately 500 miles) and keep you running in good health.

If possible, go to a running specialty store staffed by experienced runners. Visit the store in the late afternoon or evening, which is when your feet will have swelled to their longest and widest, just as they'll swell when you run. Take a pair of the socks that you wear when you run.

If you can't find a specialty store in your area, be prepared to spend even more time searching for shoes. When you find a shoe you like, insist on wearing it for a short jog down the sidewalk or in the mall corridor. Don't buy shoes from any store that won't allow you a brief tryout.

Look for shoes that fit snugly but not tightly. Too much slippage will cause blisters. Check that the toebox is roomy enough for the front of your feet.

Most shoes have either EVA or polyurethane midsoles. EVA feels softer, more flexible, and bouncier in the store, but polyurethane might be the better choice if you are a serious runner. Carbon rubber outsoles last longer than blown-rubber ones but may feel slightly harder in the store.

If you are a big runner with flat feet, you may have to worry about overpronation (your feet roll inward too much when they make contact), which can cause knee and other injuries. To see if you overpronate, place a pair of your shoes on a tabletop with the heels facing you. If the heels tilt inward a lot, you may have an overpronation problem (some pronation is normal). Motion-control shoes can reduce overpronation, and these shoes typically have wedges, bridges, or other support devices inside to stop your feet from rolling inward too far.

Once you've selected the shoes you want, give them the tabletop eyeball test as well. When new, they should stand straight and tall. You don't want to take home shoes that have a construction defect of any kind.

## ❖ Principles ❖

1. Go shoe shopping in the late afternoon or early evening, visiting (if possible) a specialty retailer whose salespeople are experienced runners with expertise in the area of running shoes. Be sure to take a short tryout jog in every shoe you're considering and take a pair of your running socks to wear.
2. Don't worry about weight. Buy the shoes that feel the best on your feet and offer the features you want.
3. Consider running in motion-control shoes if you are heavy and flat-footed. Consider cushioned shoes if you are relatively light and your feet have high arches. Otherwise, look for "stability" shoes.
4. Keep your shoes clean and dry after purchasing them, but don't toss them in the washing machine, where strong laundry detergents can affect the shoes' glues. Brush or wash your shoes clean by hand and dry them with a small fan or heat source whenever they get wet.
5. Keep track of how many miles you run in each pair of shoes. You'll need new shoes after about 500 miles.

# Apparel

Running is a four-season activity. That's one reason why it's such a health-enhancing exercise—you can do it anytime, all the time, so you don't suffer from the off-and-on yo-yo effects of other exercise routines. And it's also a big reason why runners come to appreciate the activity so much. Running through the seasons adds variety, color, and new experiences to your workouts, keeping them always different and nearly always enjoyable.

Okay, I admit it—a cold, drenching rain is not my idea of a good time. But aside from that, I enjoy running in almost all weather conditions. Summer heat isn't great for a long run, but the warm, relaxing sweat sure feels good when you limit yourself to a reasonable 30 to 40 minutes.

Spring and fall bring obvious pleasures. The smells, colors, and sounds change dramatically when nature is at her busiest. And winter, surprisingly, can be the best time of all. Every runner looks forward to the first run on a crisp, cushiony snowfall.

Dramatic improvements in running apparel have made it possible for runners to cope with just about any weather. More than cope, actually. It's now possible to run comfortably in almost all weather conditions.

The key has been the development of microfibers. These materials, which are very similar to the polyesters that were so dreaded several decades ago, allow for two key actions: They let sweat move away *from* your body, and they prevent water and wind from getting through the fibers *to* your body. The result: You stay relatively dry and cool in summer, and relatively dry and warm in winter.

In summer, you want to move sweat away from your body as rapidly as possible because evaporation cools you down. In winter, you want to produce as little of it as possible because evaporation will give you the chills. To achieve this, avoid cotton clothing and wear materials that deal more effectively with sweat.

The difference between cotton and microfibers is not a small one; it's a major one. Microfibers cost slightly more than cotton, but you get a big payoff every time you go out for a run. Most important of all, the ability to stay comfortable while running in all weather will help you stick with your program.

In winter, you need more than just a shirt, of course. You need a lightweight, breathable, windproof jacket. Again, microfibers have what you want. In most conditions, a microfiber shirt and microfiber jacket will provide all the protection you need. In frigid weather, you'll have to add another layer over both your torso (making three layers) and your legs (two layers, since your legs don't need as much). And don't forget head, ear, and hand protection. For men, the groin also needs extra protection; yes, *that* counts as an extremity, and you'll be sorry if you don't keep it warm.

## ❖ Principles ❖

1. Avoid cotton shirts and socks. Buy microfiber shirts and socks made from various polyester materials. These "wickable" materials will keep your body dry and comfortable.
2. Don't overdress in winter. You don't want to sweat profusely. If you dress just enough to stay dry, you'll also stay warm.
3. In cold weather, regulate your body temperature with a wool or microfiber cap that you can put on and take off as necessary. Chances are, you'll take it off when the wind's at your back and put it on when the wind's in your face.
4. You can also regulate your body temperature with a microfiber jacket that has a full zipper. The zipper is important, because it gives you control over the amount of air reaching your body. Zip it up tight when you're leaning into the wind, zip it down when the wind at your back warms you up.
5. In cold winter weather, always remember to cover the extremities. Your hands, ears, and groin need extra protection, particularly on windy days. Your feet usually don't.

# Heart-Rate Monitors

For many years, the only thing runners had to strap around their wrists was a watch with a sweep second hand. Now the heart-rate monitor is also competing for wrist space, and no other instrument can give you so much feedback about your workouts. That's why heart-rate monitors have proven to be so popular.

Coaches and physiologists have known for a long time that a runner's heart rate is the best measure of a workout's effectiveness, but until recently, they had no direct access to this measure. Instead, they had to grab the wrist or neck immediately after the runner stopped moving to get a manual reading.

Now, with monitors, runners have direct access to their heart rates and can even get clear and immediate feedback in the middle of a workout. The monitor can indicate whether you should run faster, run slower, or even go home to take a shower and call it a day.

There are many different ways to use a heart-rate monitor. Here are some of the key ones.

***To take your morning pulse.*** You can also do this manually, of course. The best time is just a few minutes after you have awakened, while you are still lying in bed. The idea is to keep track of your morning pulse rate so that you can spot changes quickly. When your morning pulse is elevated, you may be coming down with something or you may simply be overtraining. In either case, an elevated morning pulse tells you that you need a rest day.

***To run at your aerobic training pulse (ATP).*** This is the slowest pulse you can run at while still getting aerobic and health benefits from your workout. Your aerobic training pulse is important because it's the pace at which you should do approximately 80 percent of your weekly running, including easy days and long runs. First, you must determine your maximum heart rate, which is most simply expressed as 220 minus your age. If you're 40, your maximum heart rate is 180 ($220 - 40 = 180$).

Your ATP is 60 percent of your maximum heart rate. In the above example, the 40-year-old runner's aerobic training pulse is 108 (0.60 × 180 = 108).

By using their heart-rate monitors, many runners learn that they are training too hard much of the time. Once they learn to slow down on their aerobic training pulse runs, they recover better for other harder runs, and their fitness and vitality improve.

**To control your hard running days.** In particular, a heart-rate monitor can help you run your tempo runs and your max $VO_2$ runs at the right effort and intensity. Some runners train too fast during these workouts, just as they do on easier days. The heart-rate monitor tells them that it's okay—indeed, even preferable—to slow down.

## ❖ Principles ❖

1. A heart-rate monitor gives you direct access to the simplest, most efficient feedback tool you have: your own heart. It can help you train smarter and more scientifically than ever before.
2. Your most important heart rate is your morning heart rate. By monitoring this on a regular basis, you can determine if you are overtraining or when you might be coming down with a cold or other illness.
3. Your aerobic training pulse (ATP) is the pulse at which you should be doing approximately 80 percent of your training. Many runners train too fast most days of the week, which is wasteful and inefficient.
4. With a heart-rate monitor, you can make sure you're training at your ATP. Simply determine your maximum pulse rate (220 minus your age) and multiply it by 0.60 to get your ATP.
5. You can also use a heart-rate monitor to correctly measure the effort of your other harder training days, so you'll run at the right pace when doing tempo runs and max $VO_2$ training.

# Treadmills

For many years, most treadmills were ugly, clunky, mechanical devices that tempted few runners. By the early 1990s, however, manufacturers had awakened to the huge potential market and began making sleeker, smoother machines that suddenly made the treadmill's many advantages clear to everyone. The treadmill boom was on, and it has continued to build momentum through the years.

Many runners now consider the treadmill one of the best life-time fitness purchases they can make. While a few purists still hold treadmills in contempt, insisting that running outdoors is the only true path, most runners can see that a home treadmill offers a wonderful advantage. And when you have a treadmill, it's amazing how those occasions can add up. Cold weather. Hot weather. Rain and snow. Allergies. Darkness.

Once you start compiling the list, it grows longer and longer. Parents with young children have found that a treadmill allows them to watch their kids and get in a workout at the same time. When doing a long run, you have a ready supply of sports drinks and energy bars. Or, you can watch an instructional video or listen to language tapes while running safely on a treadmill. Some cognitive psychologists have even suggested that the mind is particularly receptive to new materials while you're running.

To buy a treadmill, visit an equipment warehouse, where you can actually run on several different models to see which you like best. Look first for stability—you don't want to be rocking and rolling while you run. Ask about the motor, to make sure it's powerful enough for the amount of running and walking you might do on it. You'll know the treadmill is powerful enough if it operates smoothly and steadily while you're running on it. The best treadmills have motors rated at 2 horsepower or greater.

Also, find out if the treadmill deck has any shock-absorbing properties. Many runners have found that they can run on a treadmill without the pain they encounter on the roads, because treadmills are softer. This is also a great way to recover from certain injuries. Note, however, that a treadmill can be *too* soft.

Running on a treadmill takes practice, but no particular skills. Start out very slowly with your normal running stride and only increase speed after you feel totally comfortable. Run at the front of the tread, where you can easily reach the controls and a bottle of sports drink (many treadmills have drink holders). When finished, get off slowly and carefully, as you may feel slightly dizzy for a moment.

Treadmills are unparalleled for hard, scientific training, since you can vary your speed precisely and monitor your heart rate at once. This gives you a chance to do great progressive workouts, in which you increase either the distance or the intensity of your run.

# ❖ Principles ❖

1. Use the treadmill to increase the frequency of your workouts. Without cold and darkness as excuses, you should be able to fit in more training and get yourself in better shape.
2. Try out several treadmills before choosing the one you like best. Pay particular attention to the smoothness and stability of the "ride." The treadmill shouldn't make you wobble from side to side or feel herky-jerky when you run on it.
3. Explore the treadmill's shock-absorbing abilities. If a treadmill lowers your risk of injury, as it should, then you have another strong reason for buying one.
4. Make sure the treadmill's top speed, and its elevation incline, are appropriate for your level. You don't want to get home and discover that you've bought a treadmill that doesn't go fast enough or has speed you can't use.
5. A treadmill can let you do the ultimate in precise training. You can know your speed and heart rate at all times, and vary them according to any formula you want to follow.

# Indoor Exercise

Treadmills are no longer the only piece of indoor exercise equipment that runners use for cross-training, easy days and foul-weather alternatives. The fitness boom has brought with it many new and improved exercise machines. When choosing one, first ask yourself: Am I doing this as a substitute for running (to improve running performance), or am I doing this as an alternative to running (for easy days and injury recovery)?

In the first case, choose a machine that mimics running as much as possible. In the latter case, where you're seeking an easy day or a workout that will help you recover from a running injury, use non-weight-bearing equipment that stresses different muscles than running. When you're injured, let pain be your guide. Only use a piece of equipment if it is not painful.

**Stationary bicycle.** Bicycling takes the weight off your legs and doesn't involve any pounding, which means that you can often bicycle even when you have a leg or foot injury (but probably not with a knee injury). To increase the value of bike training, rise out of the seat and do regular hard bursts while standing.

**Circuit training.** Circuit training refers to a workout in which you do many different exercises, mainly strength exercises, in rapid-fire succession. Not a great substitute for running, but a wonderful workout that can build your total-body fitness.

**Elliptical trainer.** The elliptical trainer is one of the newest pieces of exercise equipment and among the best for runners. Your feet and legs move in a long, gliding, elliptical motion that provides a tremendous cardiovascular and leg-strengthening workout without any pounding at all.

**Pool running.** Running without touching the ground seems ludicrous, but in fact it's one of the best alternative exercises, and several studies have also shown it to be a strong substitute as well. You need a water-running vest for flotation. Then you simply jump in, have fun, experiment, and slowly increase the intensity of your workouts.

**Rowing machine.** Rowing provides a great cardiovascular and strength workout while you're in a seated, non-weight-bearing position. Not a great substitute workout for runners, but one of the best all-around workouts to build power and fitness.

**Ski simulator.** Cross-country skiing is a great substitute for running, long practiced by many great Scandinavian runners. You should be able to ski through many injuries, as the basic motion is a pulling and gliding one, not a pounding one.

**Stairclimber.** Stairclimbers provide an excellent substitute for running, since you're lifting your legs, pushing, and carrying nearly your full body weight at all times. Don't drape yourself over the rails; use them only for balance. Maintain an upright posture and learn to step without using the rails at all, in which case you will be carrying your full body weight.

## ❖ Principles ❖

1. The wide variety of indoor exercise equipment offers many cross-training workouts. First ask yourself: Am I primarily interested in a substitute for running (to improve performance) or an alternative to running (for easy days and injury recovery)?
2. If a substitute, choose equipment that mimics running as much as possible, with leg movement, weight bearing, and a strong aerobic component.
3. Some exercise equipment requires more skill than others. Give yourself time to learn the technique, then practice. The better your technique, the more effectively you'll use the equipment.
4. If you're using equipment to recover from an injury, monitor pain levels and experiment with different machines. You should be able to find one that provides training without pain.
5. Give serious consideration to pool running. It is slow and therapeutic, and it builds strength while maintaining aerobic fitness.

Part V

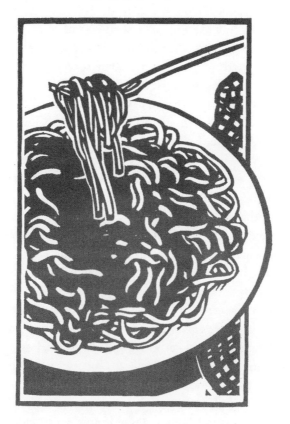

# Nutrition

# Carbohydrates

Before runners led the way to the worldwide fitness revolution, carbohydrates were largely scorned and despised. According to the then-conventional wisdom, pasta and potatoes were the poor-man's food. Worse than that, they supposedly made you fat.

Then, exercise scientists entered the picture and quickly turned everything upside down. Carbohydrates, they proved, are the best source of energy for athletes. In fact, the body prefers to burn carbohydrates before proteins and fats. In its telecast of the 1972 Olympics, ABC Sports showed Erich Segal, an ardent marathoner and its commentator for the event, eating a mountain of pancakes, just like Frank Shorter did before his gold-medal performance that day in Munich.

Since then, carbohydrates have been king. Decades of continued research have shown that for both quick and long-lasting energy, the body does indeed function more efficiently with carbohydrates than with proteins or fats.

True, if you eat too much pasta, potatoes, and pancakes, you'll gain weight. There's no getting around the calories in/calories out rule. But when you eat carbohydrate foods, the body tries really hard to burn them off when you walk, run, or simply do the housecleaning. Proteins and dietary fats are converted to body fat more easily than carbohydrates.

So runners eat carbohydrates morning, noon, and night. That's the easy part. Carbohydrates surround us in the supermarket and at home. But many of them are highly processed, sugary snacks that fall far short of the ideal because they're brimming with empty calories.

With a little effort, you can find carbohydrates that are much healthier for you. Whole-grain breads, for example, contain fiber and various vitamins and minerals. And fruits contain fiber, vitamins, and minerals not found in processed foods.

Many vegetables are also high-carbohydrate foods, though they aren't packed with enough carbos to sustain a marathoner. The vitamin and micronutrient payoff from vegetables, however, is unbeatable. That's why runners try to eat good portions of vegetables along with the pastas, rices, and other grains that often make up the main and most filling parts of their evening meals.

Since carbohydrates are burned quickly, many athletes find it a good idea to eat multiple mini-meals during the day. This practice, often called grazing, guarantees that you maintain a high energy level all day long. At the same time, since you never get hungry, you're less likely to develop a craving for an unhealthy, high-fat snack. One last benefit: Everytime you consume a meal, your body devotes calories to digesting that meal. The more meals you eat, the more calories you burn. It's like getting in extra daily workouts.

## ❖ Principles ❖

1. Make carbohydrate-packed foods the mainstay of every meal. When you run, your body burns carbohydrates more efficiently than fats or proteins. That's why marathoners carbo-load on pasta the night before a big race.
2. Eat whole-grain cereal products—wheat, rice, oatmeal, bread, bagels—to anchor each meal. These calorie-dense carbohydrate foods also contain fiber, vitamins, and minerals.
3. Consume plenty of fruits and vegetables as well. They don't provide as many calories as the cereal grains, but they are an unequaled source of vitamins, minerals, and newly discovered and extremely healthful phytochemicals.
4. Avoid empty carbohydrates, such as the ever-present snack foods, that contain excessive amounts of sugar and fat. When you have a sudden craving, select fruit or a bagel instead.
5. Consider grazing every two to three hours throughout the day rather than eating several large meals. At each mini-meal, eat some fruits, vegetables, or a low-fat protein food.

# Fats

We live in a country that is obsessed with the fat content in food. And while most people don't do a good job at limiting fats in their diets, it's smart to be concerned about them. Diets that contain too many calories and the wrong kind of fats are strongly implicated in heart disease and other lifestyle diseases such as diabetes. By changing the amount and types of fats you eat, you can substantially improve your health and running performance.

To a large extent, the type of fats seems more important than the amount. Researchers have long noted that Mediterranean peoples consume lots of fat in their diets but don't develop much heart disease. Why? Because much of the fat comes from fish oils and olive oil, a monounsaturated fat.

By contrast, people who live in countries where red meats and dairy products make up a significant part of the diet suffer from higher rates of heart disease. In this case, the culprit is saturated fats. These fats are most likely to clump together and cling to the insides of your arteries. Another fat that's fast developing a bad reputation is trans fats, partially saturated fats produced in the manufacture of processed foods ranging from chips to cakes and cookies.

Caught in the middle are the polyunsaturated fats that are present in many vegetable oils. Several decades ago, nutritionists began recommending polyunsaturated fats as a healthful alternative to saturated fats. And, indeed, they are a better alternative. But it turns out that polyunsaturated fats are only a half-step toward the preferred Mediterranean diet.

So the advice is really quite simple. Eat less red meat and whole-fat dairy products. Nutritionists suggest that you select nonfat dairy products or those with 1 percent fat contents. For salad dressings and other liquid fat needs, use olive oil or other oils high in monounsaturated fats. And eat fish several times a week.

Runners are sometimes confused by the performance aspects

of fat consumption and fat burning. Two prime examples of con-fusing advice are: (1) fats provide more calories than carbohy-drates, so fats are the best source of endurance fuel; (2) walking burns more fats than running. Both are wrong.

In a biochemical sense, fats do provide more calories per gram consumed than carbohydrates, but the running body doesn't like to burn fats for energy. It prefers carbohydrates; it uses them much more efficiently than fats. That's why runners should always eat carbohydrates before training and racing.

Second, in a given amount of time, running burns more calo-ries and more fats than walking. Your car burns more gasoline at 80 miles per hour than it burns at 40, and your body burns more fuel (including more fats) at a running pace than it burns at a walking pace. This is precisely why running is such a great weight-loss exercise.

## ❖ Principles ❖

1. Try to follow a 55-30-15 diet. That's 55 percent of calories from carbohydrates, 30 from fats, and 15 from protein.
2. Keep your consumption of fats to just 10 percent saturated fats (red meats and dairy products). Also avoid the trans fats in many processed foods like chips, cakes, and cookies.
3. Use olive oil or other monounsaturated oils, like canola oil, for salad dressings and cooking. Supplement them with the polyun-saturated fats found in many vegetable oils. Eat fish several times a week, especially cold-water fish like salmon and tuna.
4. Don't try to eliminate fats and oils from your diet. Fat is an es-sential nutrient for humans, and your body requires a modest amount of daily fat intake to maintain many important functions.
5. For maximum fat loss and weight loss, run a little faster or far-ther. Both will increase calorie and fat burning. For most run-ners, it's easier to go farther than faster, so increase the distance you run each week by no more than 10 percent.

# Proteins

Proteins are the building blocks of life, and all humans require sufficient amounts of them in their diets. But most adult Americans get far more proteins than they need, and they pay a price for it: Most of our proteins come larded with excess fat that too often contributes to weight gain, heart disease, and other lifestyle illnesses. And lest we forget, the best runners in the world hail from Kenya and Ethiopia, where the diets are notoriously low in proteins.

You might think that runners need more proteins than less-active individuals, just as they need more carbohydrates. There's not much evidence for that. In general, you'll get the extra proteins you may need simply from the extra calories you consume to maintain energy levels.

Studies have shown that runners consume more calories than non-exercisers. And in eating more foods, they also take in more key food groups and vitamins and minerals. In other words, as long as you aren't gaining weight, a high-calorie diet is most likely a healthy one because you're consuming all the nutrients you need. Running seems to point you toward the healthiest foods.

I'm assuming that you're following a reasonably well-balanced diet, with a modest number of eggs, dairy products, lean meats, fish, and fowl. A relatively high percentage of runners limit their red-meat intakes to avoid the fats that cling so closely to red meats. Even ovo-lactovegetarians or vegans (those who don't eat any eggs or dairy products) have no trouble fueling their running programs or getting enough proteins. Indeed, studies consistently find them to be extremely healthy individuals. They may, of course, need to pay more attention to the food they consume to ensure they're eating well-balanced diets.

Low-fat dairy products and fish are among the best protein sources for runners. At breakfast, many runners enjoy a small cup of low-fat, fruit-flavored yogurt—a great way to get some protein at the beginning of the day. In moderation, eggs are also an excellent protein food. The days of being obsessed about cholesterol in eggs have long since passed. It's cholesterol in our blood that contributes to heart disease risk, and blood cholesterol is much more influenced by high-saturated-fat foods like red meats and full-fat dairy products than it is by eggs.

Fish not only adds high-quality protein to your diet but also provides it in a form that lowers heart disease risk. This is very uncommon for protein foods. The heart-healthiest fish, including salmon, tuna, cod, bluefish, and other cold-water fish, contain oils that make the blood less sticky. In other words, they prevent the kind of blood clots that can lead to heart attacks. You can't go wrong by including fish in your diet two or three times a week.

## ❖ Principles ❖

1. Don't worry about proteins. Your daily diet should provide plenty, as long as it's varied and well-balanced, with occasional low-fat dairy products, eggs, lean meats, fish, and fowl.
2. Always select nonfat or low-fat (1 percent) dairy products over the higher-fat options. You'll get the same high-quality protein without the high saturated fat that can lead to heart disease.
3. When eating red meats, make careful selections at the supermarket and trim additional fat in preparation. See if you and your family can develop a taste for meat substitutes that use soy products. Soy contains isoflavones, which are thought to work as antioxidants that block cancer-causing substances.
4. Eat fish several times a week. Fish provides an excellent source of protein with fatty acids that are naturally protective against heart disease.
5. Check out various ethnic cookbooks and recipes for the healthy and flavorful ways they combine grains, nuts, seeds, and beans. In most of the world, red meat is still a luxury, yet populations everywhere find ways to meet their protein needs.

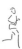

# Vitamins and Minerals

When you run and burn hundreds of extra calories every day, you can't eat the way a sedentary person eats. You have to eat better. To acquire and maintain the optimal health you're seeking, you'll certainly want to make sure you get all the necessary vitamins, minerals, and micronutrients you need.

Fortunately, this is relatively easy. As nutritional science marches forward, uncovering new and previously overlooked nutrients, an age-old truism grows stronger and stronger: Eat a varied, well-balanced diet.

Processed foods may not include all the original nutrients; they may have been destroyed in the preparation and preserving processes that are designed to increase shelf life. Pills also can't include all the nutrients; they are composed of whatever vitamins and minerals the manufacturer has chosen.

To get all the nutrients you need, you have to eat the real thing. And that means, just as your mother told you, eat your vegetables and fruits. These foods contain hundreds of recently discovered compounds that are impressing researchers with their health-enhancing and illness-preventing powers.

For runners in particular, juices are a wonderful way to consume some of your daily vegetables and fruits. Juices are great before and after a run—all day long, for that matter. They'll help keep you fully hydrated; they'll deliver a wide range of vitamins, minerals, and phytochemicals; and they'll provide some extra energy you can use during the day. Stick with 100 percent juices, and don't stop with just fruit juices. Include tomato and vegetable juices as well. In addition, don't forget to munch on the solid forms of fruits and vegetables, because they provide fiber.

In recent years, the antioxidants vitamins C and E and beta-carotene have gained strong support in several major studies, and it makes sense for runners to give special attention to these vitamins.

Vitamin C and vitamin E seem to be the most powerful. You can get plenty of vitamin C from fruit juices, and you can also supplement with little trouble. Try to get 60 milligrams per day. One cup of orange juice provides 97 milligrams of vitamin C. Vitamin E is not so easily obtained in the diet, so you'll have to turn to supplements. Try to get at least 30, but no more than 200, international units a day.

Runners may also need additional potassium and magnesium for proper electrolyte balance and muscle functioning. Bananas are a popular source of potassium, and magnesium is found in most vegetables.

The daily multivitamin remains extremely popular among runners. You can get many of the vitamins and minerals you need from a pill. To get them all, however, you need to eat the real thing—a variety of whole foods, especially fruits and vegetables.

# ❖ Principles ❖

1. For optimal nutrition, eat a varied, well-balanced diet that includes plenty of fruits and vegetables. Whole foods contain many phytochemicals and other micronutrients that can't be obtained from processed foods.
2. Drink fruit and vegetable juices as another way to tap into this powerhouse of nutrients. They'll keep you well-hydrated while also providing many vitamins and minerals.
3. To make sure you're getting all the fruits and vegetables you need, eat them as healthful snacks during the day. Fruits make an obvious snack, but crispy handfuls of carrots, celery, cucumbers, or other favorite vegetables are great desk foods.
4. Consider taking a supplement or supplements that contain the main antioxidants: vitamins C and E and beta-carotene. Vitamins C and E are especially important to runners.
5. If you feel the need for nutritional insurance, take a daily multivitamin/mineral. But don't use this as an excuse for not eating healthful whole foods during the day.

# Before and after a Run

As you get closer to a workout or race, you have to be more careful about what you eat. The last several hours are particularly important. You can make some good choices, or you can make some very bad choices—the kind that can ruin a race for which you've spent two to three months training.

After a workout or race, you could, I suppose, eat almost anything and not worry about it. Sometimes, that makes sense. After a marathon, for example, it's tempting to binge on all of the foods you've probably been keeping at arm's length for several months. Fair enough. You deserve a reward. But even then, there are compelling reasons to make intelligent food choices.

First, let's turn back to the all-important pre-run situation. What should you avoid? Foods that are likely to give you stomach or bowel problems while you're running: high-fiber foods; fruits that go right through your system; fatty, greasy foods; a last-second cup of coffee. Everyone has his own personal trouble foods. Do the commonsense thing and avoid yours before running.

If you run or race early in the morning, you won't have time to eat a substantial breakfast, but it's almost always a good idea to get some basic carbohydrates into your stomach. Try a piece of toast, a bagel, an energy bar, or a banana. A small cup of sports drink will help you get through a short run. If you're running longer, try to drink more, for both the water content and the carbohydrates.

If you're running later in the day, you should have had time for several meals to make sure your tank is full. Now, you just need to top it off a little. Consider a full glass of sports drink, especially if you haven't been paying much attention to drinking during the day. In recent years, energy bars have become an excellent and widely available choice as well as a tasty snack.

After your workout or race, the best nutrition strategy is to mirror what you did immediately before. It makes sense, doesn't it? You needed fluids and carbohydrates before your run; you sweated and burned them off while running, so now you need them again. Studies have shown that your body is most receptive to carbohydrates in the 15 to 20 minutes after you finish your run. It's also a good idea to include a little protein at this point—a glass of low-fat milk, low-fat yogurt, or a handful of nuts.

Finally, drink some water, sports drink, or fruit juice as soon as possible after your run, and then keep at it. Your thirst is not a reliable guide to your fluid needs; you need more than you think. The sooner you replenish your fluids and carbohydrates, the more energy you'll have for other activities and for your next workout.

# ❖ Principles ❖

1. Eat a light, easily digestible carbohydrate food one to two hours before you begin running or racing. Good suggestions include an energy bar, a bagel, a piece of toast and jam, or a banana.
2. Avoid foods that are likely to upset your stomach and bowel: greasy foods; certain fruits; high-fiber foods; heavy, high-protein foods; a last-minute cup of coffee.
3. Drink eight ounces of sports drink 30 minutes before you run. This will help supply both the water and the carbohydrates you need during your run.
4. After running or racing, getting rehydrated and staying hydrated should be your most important concern. Drink as soon as possible after running and several more times in the hours immediately following your workout or race. Thirst isn't a reliable guide to how much fluid you need; you should force yourself to drink more.
5. After a run, you need to consume much the same foods and fluids you ate beforehand. This is a good time to drink a fruit juice you avoided before running and also an excellent time for a light protein food like low-fat yogurt or a handful of nuts.

# On the Run

The science and practice of nutrition during a long workout or race has changed and improved so much in the last several decades that it's scarcely recognizable. When I first began running marathons in the mid-1960s, I was advised not to eat or drink anything during a race. If I did, according to the wisdom of the time, I'd get stomach cramps or side stitches. Now, runners have all manner of drinks, gels, bars, and lozenges to consume while running, and plenty of research to prove the value of such practices.

The basic idea is twofold, and the refrain is familiar. When running for more than an hour, you need to (1) rehydrate yourself on a regular basis, and (2) consume some simple carbohydrates to maintain your energy reserves. The longer you're running, the more important the fluids and carbohydrates become.

During workouts or races of less than 60 minutes, drinking and eating probably aren't so important. I say probably because some recent research has shown that consuming a sports drink during an interval-training session that lasted for less than one hour improved the quality of the session.

There's also good reason to think that fluids and carbohydrates consumed during almost any short workout or race can improve your recovery from the effort. In other words, drinking and taking in carbohydrates decrease the stresses of the workout enough to help your body bounce back quickly and be ready for the next run. Since all coaches and runners accept recovery as a key component of a training program, this is an important concept.

Still, most runners worry primarily about long runs and marathon races, and this is the area that has attracted the most attention and produced the most results.

A sports drink is your number one ally because it contains both water and simple sugars (carbohydrates) in the exact percentage that has been shown to work best in an exercising body.

According to the American College of Sports Medicine, you should consume six to eight ounces of a sports drink or water every 15 to 20 minutes during a long run or race.

Bars and gels have also become very popular among marathoners. Some runners feel that these more concentrated carbohydrates provide the bigger boost that they need late in a marathon. Be sure to wash them down with water, not with sports drink, or you could get too much sugar in your stomach.

With the growing popularity of marathons, the original energy supplement—glucose tablets—has reappeared. These are easy to use, as are other hard candies, but you should realize that they provide only small amounts of carbohydrates.

# ⬥ Principles ⬥

1. Consuming sports drinks and carbohydrates during almost any run decreases the stresses on your body and improves the post-workout recovery. Even when performance is not directly enhanced, recovering quickly from workouts is a major plus.
2. During long runs and marathons, try to take in six to eight ounces of a sports drink every 15 to 20 minutes. The commercial drinks contain just the right combination of water and sugars (carbohydrates). You don't have to worry about anything.
3. When planning long workouts, set out your drinks the night before, allow yourself time to stop briefly at a convenience store to buy a drink, carry drinks with you in a fanny pack, or run a loop course that passes your home several times.
4. Try the various bars, gels, and glucose supplements to see which work best for you. Be sure to wash them down with water. Don't try anything in a marathon if you haven't already used it in training.
5. If you have to walk briefly to consume your drinks or gels, don't worry about it. The few seconds that you lose while walking are much better than the minutes you'll lose if you hit the wall.

# Drinks, Bars, and Gels

As the worldwide running population grew to tens of millions in the last several decades, the food market responded with products designed specifically for these runners. First came the sports drinks, then energy bars, and, most recently, energy gels.

Gatorade was the first of the sports drinks, PowerBar the first of the bars, and Gu the first of the gels. Each of these has come to stand for an entire category, but each has also been joined by many competitors with similar properties.

When choosing among them, personal preference is often the best guide. That is, use the product that tastes best to you. That way, you'll use more of it, which is the idea behind these energy foods.

Of course, you could choose a bagel, a banana, or a glass of orange juice. Indeed, fruits will provide vitamins, minerals, fiber, and phytochemicals in addition to carbohydrates. But drinks, bars, and gels have two principal benefits. First, they're handily packaged, easy to transport, and designed for ease of use by runners and other active athletes.

Second, and more important, the carbohydrate formulations have been scientifically prepared to deliver the maximum amount of energy without other complications. The bars, for example, don't contain much fiber, because fiber can cause problems just before or during a workout.

The drinks are the most important of the three products, and you'd be hard-pressed to find a juice that works as well. That's because the drinks are specially formulated to deliver the maximum amount of water and carbohydrates at the same time. Most juices, colas, and other sweet beverages contain too much sugar, which is a carbohydrate that your body would normally be happy to burn.

When beverages contain too much sugar, however, they empty slowly from your stomach into your bloodstream. The result is that you don't get rehydrated quickly. Quick rehydration is the first and most important role of a sports drink. It's more important than supplying carbohydrates, because getting dehydrated is a more serious health risk than running out of carbohydrates.

In the final analysis, properly formulated sports drinks should be your first line of defense against dehydration and carbohydrate depletion. During a hard workout or race, you should consume six to eight ounces of sports drink every 15 to 20 minutes. That's quite a bit, so you'll have to make sure there's plenty available and you'll have to concentrate on drinking often.

Energy bars and gels are also great sources of readily available carbohydrates. But if you take them during a race or workout, you still have to consume the liquids. And in this case, it should be just water. If you drink a sports drink with a bar or gel, you'll push the sugar concentration in your stomach too high, slowing the fluid's absorption into your bloodstream.

# ❖ Principles ❖

1. When you're running hard or racing, your body needs up to eight ounces of water every 15 to 20 minutes, plus 10 to 15 grams of carbohydrate energy (40 to 60 calories).
2. Commercial sports drinks contain a special formulation with the scientifically correct ratio of sugars to water. Many other drinks, from juices to colas, contain too much sugar, which slows the absorption of water into the bloodstream. Since quick rehydration is the first and most important role of a sports drink, choose the sports drinks for their special formulations.
3. Bars and gels also contain excellent carbohydrates, but you still need to get that all-important water every 15 to 20 minutes.
4. When taking bars and gels, don't consume sports drinks at the same time. Wash them down with water and nothing else.
5. For maximum exercise results, buy bars and gels that provide a high-carbohydrate formulation rather than high-protein or "40-30-30" formulations.

# Vegetarian Diet

Many people decide to make major dietary changes when they begin running programs or increase their commitments to healthy fitness lifestyles. They figure it makes little sense to improve their exercise regimen without also improving their nutrition. And they're right.

A vegetarian diet is particularly popular. There are far more vegetarians among runners than among the general population. Perhaps it's because both follow simple, basic paths to a given end.

When I first tried a vegetarian diet three decades ago, I was worried that it wouldn't provide enough raw fuel for my then-high-mileage training program. After all, most other athletes were still eating all the steak they could gobble down. I felt drawn to the ethical, ecological, and nutritional arguments for vegetarianism, but I also wanted to be the best runner I could be.

I read everything I could find at the time—not much—and before long, I had fashioned a healthy, energy-packed vegetarian diet (technically ovo-lactovegetarian, since I ate dairy products and the occasional egg) that worked well for me. In the last 30 years, much more has been learned about the benefits—and a few risks—of the vegetarian diet. In fact, studies have consistently shown that vegetarians live longer and healthier lives than meat-eaters do, though there are several possible explanations for this outcome.

It is also now known that vegetarian runners have trained and competed successfully at the highest levels of the sport. If you're interested in pursuing this diet, here's what you need to understand about several key nutritional concerns.

***Carbohydrates.*** Vegetarians do fine here as long as they put rice, pasta, potatoes, breads, and a whole range of grains at the core of their diets. These grains, which should be included in every meal, also provide plenty of fiber, one of the things that makes vegetarian eating so healthy.

**Proteins.** Many people worry that they won't get enough proteins if they follow vegetarian diets, but this is rarely an issue. Vegans—those who don't eat eggs or dairy products—have to be a little more careful, but even they find it easy to get enough proteins if they regularly consume nuts and seeds along with plenty of soybean products and other beans. Ovo-lactovegetarians easily meet their protein needs with small portions of dairy foods and eggs.

**Fats.** Vegetable and cooking oils make it easy for vegetarians to get sufficient fats in their diets. However, ovo-lactovegetarians should avoid excessive use of creamy salad dressings and dairy products, which are high in saturated fats.

**Vitamins and minerals.** Vegetarian diets can be low in vitamin $B_{12}$, vitamin D, iron, and zinc. Supplements are a good alternative, or you can be scrupulous about getting plenty of enriched soy products, wheat germ, and dark green leafy vegetables.

## ❖ Principles ❖

1. While not for everyone, the vegetarian diet has proven very successful for some runners. It has the same pure and simple appeal as running itself.

2. Studies show that vegetarian diets can be extremely healthy, perhaps because vegetarians eat ample amounts of fresh fruits and vegetables. Runners will also have to concentrate on getting plenty of carbohydrates.

3. Ovo-lactovegetarians can easily get enough proteins by eating regular small portions of eggs and low-fat dairy products. Vegans should consider regular use of soybean products. They should also combine grains, beans, and seeds or nuts in the same meal.

4. Be careful about fats, not because you won't get enough of them but because you could get too much.

5. If you feel the need for added assurance, take a daily vitamin-mineral supplement. Of particular importance to vegetarians are vitamins $B_{12}$ and D, iron, and zinc.

# Part VI

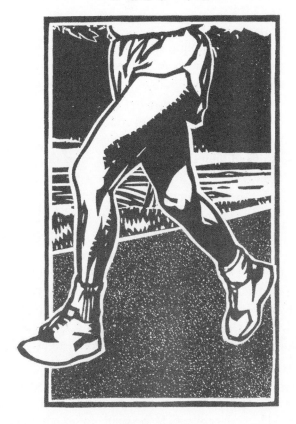

# Training

# Warming Up
## and Cooling Down

Warming up and cooling down are two of the oldest and most traditional running practices. It's easy to understand the logic behind both. The warmup literally warms up the body, preparing it for anything from a casual jog to the Olympic final.

To train or race without warming up would be like rolling out of bed in the morning and hitting the ground running (literally). You'd be so stiff and tight that you wouldn't enjoy the experience or perform well.

A well-orchestrated warmup, on the other hand, loosens your legs and the rest of your body. When you're finished, you'll actually feel a rising energy. You'll want to run. Just as important, you'll be ready to perform with maximum efficiency.

The cooldown may take place after a workout or race, but its purpose is to prepare you for the upcoming hours or days before your next workout. The goal for that time period is to help your body recover and regenerate for your next run. A cooldown assists in this process. Skip the cooldown, and you risk tightness or injury that could interfere with future workouts.

Most of your warmup, which should last from 5 to 60 minutes, should take the form of light jogging, massaging, and stretching, which should be very gentle. (The best time to stretch thoroughly is during your cooldown.) If you're warming up for a typical relaxed five-mile run, you don't have to do anything but start slowly. You can also start with a minute or two of walking before breaking into a run.

Another great routine is to stop after five minutes of running to do a little self-massage and stretching. This go-stop-go pattern can be annoying to some, though.

Before a race or a speed workout, you should take the time for a more thorough warmup that includes periods of relaxation mixed with more intense running, with the two building toward the race's start. Your prerace warmup should include a number of strides at race pace to accustom your body to the race effort. Follow the strides with easy jogging until the race begins.

Research shows that it's best, at this point, to keep moving. Don't sit or lie down. Even when you're on a crowded start line, keep jogging lightly in place.

The cooldown is the best time for more thorough stretching. Your body is fully loose and ready to be put through a routine of unforced stretching that can keep joints and muscles healthy and supple. This is also a great time for some vigorous self-massage to work out the kinks.

# ◈ Principles ◈

1. The warmup prepares your body for a workout or race. The cooldown prepares it for the recovery period that follows a run. Different roles, both important.
2. The key to a successful warmup is a gradual increase in the intensity of movement. Begin by walking, then jog, then run a little harder, then do some sprints. There's always a sense of building toward the moment of release—the start.
3. Even when you're on the start line, keep jogging lightly in place. Studies show that this will keep you fully tuned up for the start.
4. The key to a successful cooldown is simply to do it. Too many runners, in a rush to return to their many responsibilities, skip the cooldown. At the very least, reward yourself with several minutes of soothing self-massage and stretching.
5. Stretching is far better performed during the cooldown than during the warmup. Your body is more prepared for the stretches after a race or workout, so you can do them more effectively and with less risk of injury.

# Hard and Easy Workouts

The stresses involved with supporting and moving your body weight over considerable distances burn calories and strengthen your heart, but they also take a toll on your muscles and connective tissues. As a result, top coaches and physiologists realized long ago that runners must follow a hard-day/easy-day program.

At its simplest, this means that you should follow every day of hard training with an easy recovery day. A recovery day can be a day off, a day of easy jogging, or a day of strength training and other cross-training exercises.

Understanding the hard/easy principle is more important than following an exact schedule. In other words, to avoid injuries and burnout, you must respect the various stresses associated with hard training. You must learn to listen to your body and all the early warning signals it gives you, varying from an elevated morning pulse to muscle soreness and general fatigue.

In practice, many runners, even elite runners, take more than one easy day after each hard day. The ratio is more like one hard to two easy, or even up to one to four. Others prefer to think of weeks of training at a time, so they follow a two-to-five schedule, with two hard days and five easy days in a week. The numbers are less important than an appreciation for the general rule.

The hard/easy principle also extends to longer periods of time. Top runners worldwide take one to two easy months at the end of each year, during which they recover and re-energize after a long season of training and racing. I personally believe that it's a good idea to take one easy week per month, particularly when you're in a serious buildup phase, perhaps preparing for a marathon.

The easy days and weeks have two main purposes. First, they help you avoid injuries, the main bugaboo in any running program. If you can stay injury-free, you can keep training as you planned, maximizing your chances for success.

Second, the easy days have a direct, positive impact on your fitness because your body actually grows stronger when given the chance to adapt to workouts. Successive hard workouts only serve to overload your muscles and cause fatigue. It takes a rest period between workouts to give your body the chance to recover, adapt, and grow stronger.

So what's a hard workout? That is the key question. The answer: any workout that's longer or faster than your typical workout. Plus, any other workout that you do while unusually taxed by a cold, a long travel day, a fight with your boss/wife/child, or any of a thousand other stresses.

When in doubt, err on the side of caution. This is probably one of the most important ideas in running. Because running is, by its nature, such strenuous exercise, you don't have to worry much about getting enough hard days. The mistake you have to avoid is doing too many hard days.

# ❖ Principles ❖

1. Alternate hard training days with easy training days. For most runners, the ratio shouldn't be one to one but one to three or even one to four. Give your body plenty of time to adapt to each hard workout and grow stronger before the next hard workout.
2. A hard workout is one that's longer or faster than your typical daily workout. If you're not sure, err on the side of caution.
3. An easy day can be a day off, a day of easy jogging, a day of walking, or a day of strength training and other cross-training.
4. Heed the many warning signs that sometimes tell you to take an easy day or, more likely, a week of easy days. These include sore muscles, an elevated morning pulse, lethargy, slight cold-like symptoms, difficulty sleeping, and loss of appetite.
5. When training hard, consider taking an easy week every month. Always take several easy weeks at the end of the year to reward yourself for a successful year.

# Progressive Training

Sometimes, the best training system is the simplest system, and that's what progressive training is. The way I define it, progressive training is training that takes a basic workout and repeats it over and over again, increasing either the distance or the intensity of the workout (or, in a few instances, both).

Progressive training is what all beginners do. Ditto for marathoners. Beginners walk and run, then walk a little less and run a little more. Marathoners concentrate on trying to build up the distance of their long runs, mile by mile, week by week.

Progressive training has many other applications as well. You can use it to increase your speed (with intervals), your leg strength (with hill workouts), or your abs strength (with situps and crunches).

The beauty of progressive training is its simplicity. Every progressive-training plan involves increasing the time or distance run; increasing the number of pickups, intervals, or repeats; increasing speed; or decreasing rest periods. You select the one you want and develop a workout plan for the next five to six weeks.

It's important to note that, because these workouts are progressing, some ingredient is always changing. It's getting longer or faster. Or, in the case of rest periods, it's getting shorter. Progressive workouts are the sworn enemy of static programs, complacency, and laziness. That's one reason why they're so successful.

Progressive workouts are also easy to monitor and measure. Everything goes by the numbers. Some runners will find this intimidating, but they shouldn't. A good progressive-training plan, like any other plan, has to be doable. And you'll get a real sense of accomplishment as you complete each one.

It's very important to note that progressive training isn't something you do every day. Usually, do it once a week, concentrating on a particular type of workout, like speed or a long run.

You could have two series of progressive workouts paralleling each other. On Wednesdays, for example, you could run 400-meter repeats, adding one per week. On Sundays, you could do long runs, adding a mile per week. But, since progressive workouts are hard days, do them no more than twice a week.

I don't recommend doing a series of progressive-training workouts for more than about six weeks. Push on farther than that, and you're likely to get stale.

You can, however, build six weeks of one type of progressive training on top of six weeks of another type. For example, you can follow six weeks of long, easy runs with six weeks of hill training and then six weeks of speedwork. This is a very popular combination that has been proven by the success of thousands of runners.

# ❖ Principles ❖

1. Progressive training is the simplest and one of the most effective types of training. Progressive workouts follow a repetitive pattern, getting longer or faster every week.
2. An example is to run at a steady pace for 18 minutes, then turn back. On the return, run fast for 1 minute out of every 3. The next week, run 21 minutes before turning back and beginning the fast runs. The third week, run 24 minutes and turn back.
3. Another example is to run 4 laps on a track, sprinting the straightaways and jogging the curves. The next week, run 5 laps, with the same sprint/jog pattern. Repeat the workout pattern once a week until you are covering 10 laps.
4. Do a workout from one progressive-training series just one day a week, or add a second progressive workout from a different series. Continue your progressive-training series for no longer than six weeks before you take a rest or switch to a different series.
5. In general, organize your progressive-training series so that you do slow, long-distance training, followed by hill work, followed by tempo training, followed by shorter workouts that emphasize a faster pace.

# Hills

Long before the advent of modern-day sports, running hills was one of the most efficient ways to train, and that fact has not changed to this day. In ancient times, the nomadic peoples of East Africa trekked up and down the hills of the 2,000-mile-long Rift Valley. Little has changed over the millennia, and today Kenya and Ethiopia produce a spectacularly disproportionate number of the world's best distance runners.

Hill training ranks among the best training for three basic reasons, one of them less obvious than the others. Climbing hills is hard work and tests both the heart (cardiovascular training) and the legs (strength training). You can't get a better combination.

Running uphill also lessens the impact force of each footfall. Impact force is a major contributor to the overuse injuries that trouble many runners. This means that there is less risk to training hard on the hills several times a week than there is to training hard on a track or other surface. Many coaches and distance runners realize this and use hill training to great benefit. (Be careful running downhill, as this increases impact force and injury potential.)

As with any kind of new workout, you should begin hill training easily and gradually. The simplest hill workout is a medium-distance run that includes several good hills on the route. If you live in a suburban neighborhood with many roads, you could find a hilly street and loop up it several times on your run.

For more specific hill training, do hill repeats. First, find a hill that's 100 to 200 meters long on a wide road in an area that doesn't have much traffic. You don't want to be worried about cars while you're running hills.

On your first day of hill repeats, do just three or four. Run the hill at a strong, steady pace, but don't try to sprint. Good hill-running form includes a short, quick stride with moderate knee lift. Don't overstride or exaggerate the knee lift. Pump your arms forcefully to help drive yourself forward and upward. Picture a steam locomotive chugging up a hill, and chug along yourself.

At the top of the hill, turn and jog very slowly and carefully to the bottom, being careful about the impact force mentioned above. Repeat this workout once a week until you have run 10 hard efforts up the hill. Then take a rest from hill training for several weeks or months, depending on your schedule.

Most coaches and running programs advise that a hill-training phase of three to six weeks should be followed by three to six weeks of interval and speed training as you get closer to the event where you want to produce a peak effort. Hill training builds strength and power, the foundation for faster running. But it also saps the legs, so don't do it too close to any important races.

## ❖ Principles ❖

1. Hill training is an extremely versatile and efficient part of any running program. It helps build cardiovascular and leg strength, with minimal risk of injury. (Just be careful about downhill running, which increases the potential for injury.)
2. It's easy to include simple hill training in your medium and long runs. If you want, you can even push the hills while maintaining a steady effort on the downhills and flats.
3. Specific hill training requires that you find a hill that's 100 to 200 meters long. Run it at a hard but controlled effort just three or four times the first week. Jog down gently to avoid the impact force. Continue running hill repeats once a week, adding 1 additional repeat per week until you have reached 10 repeats.
4. Follow three to six weeks of hill training with a phase of three to six weeks of intervals and speed training. Don't do any hillwork at this point. Allow your legs to freshen up and get faster.
5. Even when you're not training for a particular race, make moderate hill training a regular part of your running. No other training produces as many good effects.

# Cross-Training

Once upon a time, about 20 years ago to be precise, runners believed they didn't have to do anything but run. They figured that they only had so many training minutes in a day and no time to waste. Exercise physiologists even had a phrase to support this belief—"specificity of training."

This meant, loosely, that if you wanted to be good at water polo, you'd better have spent all of your time practicing water polo; and if you wanted to be good at running, you'd better have spent all of your time running. Any other kind of training wasn't specific enough to the muscles of your desired sport to do much good.

The specificity-of-training rule still stands to a large degree, only now it's interpreted more flexibly than before. Yes, runners had better make sure that the lion's share of their training is spent on running. But there are many good reasons to practice other activities as well—to do cross-training, that is—even if you don't get an immediate payback from the stopwatch.

The best and most important reason is injury prevention. The specificity of running means that it stresses the same muscles over and over again, sometimes to the point of breakdown.

Cross-training gives those muscles a rest while building others. The end result is that you develop a more coordinated, more balanced body. This should eventually produce better racing times because you'll get injured less frequently. And consistent training is essential if you want improved performances.

Cross-training also adds variety and motivation to a training program. This is probably more important to recreational runners than to Olympic aspirants, who get plenty of motivation from their nightly dreams about gold medals. Less inspired runners, including the vast majority of us, often find that they need some variety and excitement to get pumped up for their next workouts.

Cross-training can provide that. One day you run, the next

day you bike or hit the strength room or swim. The goal isn't to win the Ironman Triathlon but to keep motivation high while achieving full-body fitness.

This isn't to imply that you must do all forms of cross-training in order to get any benefit. Many runners simply run and lift weights. Others enjoy bicycling or pool running.

Still others branch off in different directions: cross-country skiing, the martial arts, soccer. Cross-training has no limits; that's its beauty and intent. You can run as your primary fitness activity and add whatever other sports and activities you enjoy the most.

A final reason to cross-train: It burns calories, no matter what activities you choose.

# ❖ Principles ❖

1. For a variety of reasons, cross-training can be a valuable addition to your training program. The specificity-of-training rule argues that cross-training won't make you faster, but common sense and real-life practice argue that it makes many contributions to your overall health and fitness.
2. Cross-train to prevent injuries and recover from them. Cross-training develops a variety of muscles, while running tends to stress the same muscles over and over again.
3. For runners, the following cross-training activities, in descending order of benefit, will contribute the most to your running performances: elliptical-trainer workouts, bicycling, pool running, cross-country skiing, weight training. Give these priority.
4. Because it offers so much variety, cross-training can help you stay motivated and stick with your exercise program. You don't have to do the same thing day after day. You can play with a wide variety of exercise options.
5. Cross-training helps you burn more calories without increasing your risk of injury. This keeps you in shape and allows you to do harder training on those days when you run.

# Groups

For too many years, people thought of running as a lonely, individualistic sport. This resulted from two things. First, until the mid-1970s, running barely existed as a fitness sport. It was a competitive sport, and the few people who pursued it were strong-willed individualists. Second, a cult book and movie, *Loneliness of the Long Distance Runner*, provided an apt phrase to describe runners at the time.

Today, many, if not most, runners work out in groups or at least with a training partner. A partner can provide so much to make your running more enjoyable and more productive. Motivation. Fun. Better speedwork. Easier long runs. These are just a few of the reasons for group running.

Motivation is probably the biggest. When you know someone else is going to meet you somewhere at a pre-arranged time, you feel a responsibility to be there. The other person is counting on you. So you make running a priority and get there for the workout. When you run by yourself, you often fail to make it a priority, and then the opportunity to run can slip by before you realize it.

Partners also make running more fun. Because 80 to 90 percent of running is done at an aerobic pace, even among Olympic-caliber athletes, you have plenty of opportunity to shoot the breeze. You could talk on any other occasion, of course, but most people don't set aside time just for chatting. The socializing is an added benefit and often a big one. Getting in touch with others makes you feel good.

Speedwork is much easier to do with a partner or group than alone. Just as bikers benefit from drafting behind a pack of riders, you'll find it less physically and mentally strenuous to do fast training with a pack of other runners. That's why most of the world's great runners have developed from clubs or teams that trained together. The same is true for long runs. If you know you're going to be joining a couple of friends, a two- to three-hour run is something you'll actually look forward to.

Group running does have its pitfalls, nonetheless. It's imperative that you find training partners at your ability level. Otherwise, you'll have to run too hard or too slowly. You'll know you're running too hard when you can't pass the talk test. That is, you can't carry on a normal conversation during the run. Another good time for solo running is when you're working on your form and don't want to be distracted by anyone else.

Still, group running has much to recommend it. Even if you can only get together with someone else once a week, that's likely to provide the motivation to keep you going all week long.

## ◈ Principles ◈

1. Find an occasional or regular training partner—or group—and run with your partner whenever possible. It is very important that your partner have the same relative ability and can run at the same pace as you.
2. Hook up with a partner for your long runs. These will go much more easily—you'll actually look forward to them—if you have someone to shoot the breeze with for a couple of hours.
3. A partner or group is also very helpful when you're doing speedwork or tempo work. See if you can find a group—many clubs and companies have them—that gathers once a week for group speedwork. You'll be amazed at how much you improve in a couple of weeks.
4. A good-size group includes two to four other people. More than that, and it will be hard for everyone to tune in to the group's pace and conversation.
5. Use the talk test. If you can't carry on a normal conversation while you're running, you're straining too hard. You'll either have to get your partners to slow down or you'll have to find another group.

# Long Runs

The weekly long run should be part of every runner's training program, even if you're not building up to a marathon. Long runs improve aerobic capacity and fat-burning ability and increase weight loss and musculoskeletal strength. And you don't need to cover 20 miles at a time.

Basically, a long run is any workout that's 50 percent longer than your average run. If you typically run three miles three times a week, then, yes, a five-miler would be a long run. It wouldn't provide all the benefits just mentioned, but it would head you in the right direction and could certainly serve as a springboard to other longer efforts.

Since long runs concentrate on distance covered, you don't have to worry about speed. It's irrelevant. Many runners who don't have a lot of natural speed find this encouraging. If they have the discipline to work on their long runs, they'll be able to increase them to the desired goal distance.

If you feel like taking short walking breaks every once in a while in the middle of a long run, that's fine. Just keep moving, and keep returning to a relaxed run. When you're finished, you will have completed a perfectly acceptable training run and perhaps done it in a way that minimizes fatigue and risk of injury.

For those looking for more pacing advice—how fast should I go on my long runs?—here are some guidelines. Novice marathoners who are planning to finish their races in four hours or slower can probably run training efforts of up to 20 miles at or close to their marathon goal paces.

More experienced and faster marathoners should do their long runs anywhere from 30 seconds per mile to 90 seconds per mile slower than their marathon goal paces. If you're one of these talented athletes, you're already covering most of your training miles at a reasonably fast pace. When you step up to long runs, you need to slow down to go far enough and to avoid over-stressing your body.

Long runs are easier to do with a training partner, so find one if you can, but make sure the person's running pace is totally compatible with your own. You don't want someone pushing you to go faster during your long runs. If you can't find the right person, do the long runs alone. They won't be quite as much fun, but running at your own pace is absolutely essential.

Lastly, long runs require lots of patience. Success will surely come to those who give it time. You shouldn't increase the length of your long runs by more than 1 mile per effort, and you should do just two long runs per month once they extend beyond 10 miles (you can repeat shorter long runs once a week).

## ❖ Principles ❖

1. Do long runs (50 percent longer than your average run) to increase aerobic capacity, fat-burning ability, weight loss, and musculoskeletal strength.
2. Don't worry about speed. Keep all runs slow and relaxed. If necessary, take a 1-minute walking break every 5 to 10 minutes. Just keep moving. The goal is simply to stay on your feet for a given period of time.
3. Try to find a compatible training partner to do long runs with you. The miles will pass more easily. But don't run with someone who wants to go faster than you do. Running at your own best, most comfortable pace is essential.
4. Build up the distance of your long runs by just 1 mile per week. Patience, patience, patience. Once you've exceeded 10 miles, run long runs just once every two weeks.
5. Whenever possible, run on soft surfaces like grass and trails. As your long-run distance increases, pay more attention to the foods and fluids you consume before, during, and after your workout.

# Tempo Training

Tempo training is the most scientifically valid, proven, and effective form of training for running. Virtually unknown until the mid-1980s, it quickly became a major staple in every serious runner's training program. Best of all, it works for beginning and intermediate runners, too.

Basically, tempo training refers to running at a pace that's just a little bit slower than your 10-K race pace. Let's say that you can run a 10-K at 8-minutes-per-mile pace. In a tempo-training workout, you'd run two to four miles at about 8:20 pace.

Tempo training succeeds for several different reasons. On a purely individual basis, you determine the speed at which you run tempo workouts, because they're based on your own 10-K race pace. Because tempo training feels easier than racing, it's often described as a hard-but-controlled pace. Tempo workouts don't force you to strain, and they're easy to recover from.

Physiologists like tempo training because it has been shown to increase your lactate-threshold running speed. That means that you improve your ability to run fast without accumulating lots of lactic acid in your muscles. Lactic acid produces the burn and fatigue in your muscles when you are working them hard.

As lactic acid builds up, it lowers your ability to run efficiently and eventually forces you to slow down. When you raise your lactate threshold, you can run farther and faster before you hit the point where your leg-muscle contractions begin to slow down.

Some runners, particularly marathoners, like to do their tempo training as part of their medium-long runs. For example, in the middle of a relaxed 12-mile run, you do 4 hard-but-controlled miles at tempo-training pace.

Others prefer to do lactate-threshold training as part of an interval-training session on a track or trail, and this works fine, too. Run repeats of 800 meters to 1 mile at your tempo pace, taking short jogging breaks of two to four minutes between repeats. Don't run repeats that are shorter than 800 meters, and aim for a total of 2 to 4 miles worth of repeats per workout (that is, do anything from 4 × 800 to 4 × 1 mile).

Don't do more than four miles of hard running in any tempo-training workout, and don't do tempo training more than once a week. The beauty of the program is the hard-but-controlled pace. As soon as you do too much tempo training or repeat it too often, you lose the control and, therefore, the effectiveness of the training.

It's far better to integrate tempo training into a well-rounded program that also includes hill training, speedwork, and longer running. When you do, you'll see the results of your tempo training in as little as three weeks.

## ❖ Principles ❖

1. Tempo training is the single most effective form of training for runners. Its success stems from its basis as a hard-but-controlled workout. This guarantees that it produces a strong training effect without overly fatiguing you.
2. Tempo-training workouts are run at a pace that is 10 to 30 seconds slower than your best 10-K racing pace (10 for faster runners, 30 for slower runners), and include two to four miles of running at this pace. Don't run more than four miles at tempo pace in any one workout.
3. You can run your tempo workouts as hard, steady efforts in the middle of a longer run (4 miles in the middle of a 12-miler) or as interval-training repeats of 800 meters to 1 mile.
4. Don't run tempo workouts more than once a week. If you do, you risk overtraining because you lose the "controlled" part of the workout and begin to accumulate too much fatigue.
5. As your fitness improves, you can increase the pace of your tempo runs. But make them realistic for your present condition. Don't base them on your dream condition and risk overtraining.

# Max VO$_2$

All aerobic endurance activities, like running, bicycling, swimming, and cross-country skiing, are essentially contests to see how much oxygen your body can deliver to your exercising muscles. Increase the amount of oxygen, and you can run, bike, swim, or ski faster.

In running, of course, those muscles are in your legs. As you train, two things happen to improve your muscles' ability to use oxygen. First, your heart gets stronger and delivers more oxygen; and second, your leg muscles get better at using the oxygen.

In their laboratory research, scientists frequently measure this delivery and use of oxygen, calling it maximum oxygen uptake or VO$_2$ max. They consider maximum oxygen uptake to be the most basic measure of aerobic fitness, and they've shown that it increases as you train more and harder. I generally reverse the letter order, since max VO$_2$ has a friendlier sound than VO$_2$ max.

As your aerobic capacity increases, you can run farther and faster. All training improves your aerobic capacity, even slow, relaxed jogging. But some workouts improve it more than others.

The best and most efficient way to increase your aerobic capacity is to run slightly faster (10 to 30 seconds per mile) than your 5-K race pace. Faster runners should be closer to the 10-second figure, and slower runners closer to the 30-second figure. For example, if you can race a 5-K at 7:40 per mile, you should run your max VO$_2$ workouts at 7:20 to 7:30 pace. This isn't a pace that you can maintain very long in training. You can run for distance (800 meters) or time (3 to 5 minutes).

After each repeat, jog for four to five minutes, and then do another. The workout is finished when you've completed three to four repeats (for beginning and intermediate runners) or six to eight repeats (for advanced runners).

Many runners do max VO$_2$ workouts on the track as part of

their interval training routines because they like to measure the lengths and times of the repeats exactly. That's fine, but it isn't necessary. You can also do max $VO_2$ workouts on a good trail, a grassy field, or any other smooth surface that allows you to run at a fast clip without fear of ankle turns. Use your watch to time the four-minute repeats, and run at a strong and fast (but not all-out) effort.

Don't do these aerobic-capacity workouts more than once a week, and skip them on weeks when you have races. These workouts cover less distance than tempo workouts, but they're more taxing because the pace is considerably harder. If you were to do several max $VO_2$ workouts a week or include one in your training program during the week of a race, you might soon find your race performances deteriorating because you'd be too fatigued to race at full strength.

# ❖ Principles ❖

1. Maximum oxygen uptake, or max $VO_2$, is a scientific measurement of the amount of oxygen your body can deliver from your heart and use in your major exercising muscles. As you get fitter, your maximum oxygen uptake increases.
2. All running increases your aerobic capacity, but the most efficient workouts for increasing it are those in which you run slightly faster than your 5-K race pace. For example, run $4 \times 800$ meters at 10 to 30 seconds per mile faster than your 5-K race pace. Jog for four to five minutes between repeats.
3. You can also run aerobic-capacity workouts off the track by running hard and fast (but not all-out) for three to five minutes at a time. Jog for four to five minutes between repeats.
4. Do aerobic-capacity training only once a week, and skip it on a week when you have a race. Otherwise, you risk overtraining and increasing your fatigue rather than your performance.
5. After six weeks of max $VO_2$ training, take a break from it for four weeks. Concentrate instead on longer, more relaxed runs.

# Speed-Form Training

The purpose of speed-form training is to improve your leg turnover (or stride frequency, as some call it), power, running economy, and relaxation while running. The best way to achieve all this is through a variety of speed drills that you run faster than the workouts in the previous chapters.

While tempo repeats last up to 20 minutes and max $VO_2$ repeats last 4 to 5 minutes, speed-form repeats should last just 30 to 60 seconds. When measuring by distance on a track, I've always found that 200 meters is a good length for speed repeats.

You should run these repeats at about the same pace you could run in a one-mile race. Since the 200-meter repeats represent only one-eighth of the mile distance, you should be able to run these hard and fast but without straining. Another way to figure your pace is to run your 5-K race pace minus 30 to 40 seconds per mile (for faster runners) or 40 to 60 seconds per mile (for slower runners).

Either way, you should be able to complete six to eight repeats of 200 meters at this pace. Take a two- to four-minute recovery jog after each repeat, before beginning the next one. While running, concentrate on feeling smooth, powerful, relaxed, and controlled. Don't overstride and don't pump your arms excessively.

Strides offer another way to work on your speed and form. While the above workout is essentially an interval workout, with its mix of faster and slower running on a track or other good surface, strides are less structured. You can do them almost anytime, anywhere. They take only a few minutes at the end of a workout.

Basically, strides are gradual accelerations over 60 to 80 meters. By running four to six strides several times a week, you help your legs and the rest of your body remember what it's like to run fast. Without strides or some type of speed-form drill, it's easy to get sloppy in your running and do only slow running with bad form (for more information, see "Good Form" on page 12). You can find yourself slipping into a pattern where you're training to run slowly and inefficiently rather than faster and more economically.

Here's how to do strides. Finish your workout, stretch for 5 to 10 minutes, and then find a smooth, level place to run (a grassy field is excellent). Lean into your first stride as you would the beginning of a race, and continue accelerating for 60 to 80 meters. Concentrate on your form, staying smooth and strong (but not straining) as you accelerate. As you reach about 90 percent of your top speed, relax and allow your body to decelerate. Jog for a minute or two, and then repeat another four or five times.

Regular doses of speed-form training are like regular tune-ups of your car engine. The car can keep running without the tune-ups, but it won't run as smoothly and efficiently as you'd like.

# ❖ Principles ❖

1. Regular speed-form training will improve your speed, power, relaxation at faster speeds, and running economy. Without it, your form will tend to get sloppy and deteriorate.
2. A good speed-form workout is to run 6 × 200 meters once every week or two at approximately the pace you could run your fastest mile. Concentrate on controlled speed during these 200-meter repeats. Don't strain. Don't overstride.
3. You can also improve your speed-form, in a less rigorous way, by running strides once or twice a week after your workout. They only take five or six gradual accelerations of 60 to 80 meters. Run strong but relaxed.
4. Other running drills can also improve your leg power and running efficiency. Among them: bounding, with long, exaggerated strides; high knees, in which you move forward very slowly but with very rapid and high knee lifts; and hot feet, or running with very fast, very short strides that improve your leg turnover.
5. Speed-form training takes only a small time commitment while yielding potentially dramatic results.

# Burnout

All training theory rests on a simple foundation—the principle of gradual adaptation to stress—that can be tauntingly difficult to follow in practice. This book contains many words to guide you toward a sound training program, one you can change and adjust to your own needs. But you may still fall into the overtraining trap.

Why? Primarily because runners are sometimes so motivated, so dedicated, and so focused on a goal that they don't follow the old adage "Listen to your body." Sure, you've had a long week of business travel or a sick child at home or exams to study for or a developing sniffle. But your program calls for a Sunday morning long run, and darn it, you're going to stick to the program.

Most of the time, such dedication pays dividends. If you don't have it, you won't succeed in reaching your goals. But you must also realize the opposite: Too much dedication can sometimes interfere with your plans. The key is to find the right balance.

To balance your training with your life, you must observe a number of physiological and commonsense principles. First, when your body is rebelling, listen to it and take it easy. Leg soreness means something. So do other aches, pains, and fever. Listen to them.

Strangely enough, there's a thin line between peak condition and burnout. Many runners fall into the burnout trap just when things are starting to go particularly well. You feel great, you're running fast, and every workout seems easy. No wonder you're tempted to run a little farther and harder every day. You sense that you're on the verge of a breakthrough.

This is often when the breakdown occurs instead. One morning, you wake up feeling sluggish and feverish. That day's run is a disaster. So are the next day's and the one after that. Concerned that you've had three or four bad days in a row, an alarm goes off in your head: You're getting out of shape!

So you push yourself really hard for the next several days, eager to have rewarding workouts. You succeed, to a point, but it takes tremendous effort. In fact, it increases your overall burnout, and soon the downward spiral continues.

When this happens, the only way out is to take several weeks, sometimes more, of rest and very easy running. You will bounce back because your body is programmed to repair itself and recover, but it won't happen as fast as you'd like.

It's far better to avoid burnout in the first place. Use common sense in your training; do less when you're facing unusual, outside stresses. And make sure that you have regular recovery days and recovery weeks built into your training program. The only way to maintain optimal fitness and energy is to give yourself appropriate breaks when you need them.

## ❖ Principles ❖

1. Listen to your body. When it's unusually tired, achy, sore, feverish, or fatigued, give yourself several rest days. Don't "push through" to make yourself tougher and stronger. It won't work.
2. Use a training program in which a hard training day is generally followed by two easy ones. Elite runners try to follow a hard-day/easy-day schedule, but most recreational athletes need an additional day of rest or recovery running.
3. At three or four key points during the year, allow yourself several weeks of easy training, perhaps after a marathon, during the hottest days of summer, or while you're on vacation. No one should train hard 52 weeks a year.
4. Don't substitute a cross-training workout for a running workout and think that you're giving yourself a rest day. It's a good idea in principle, but if you're training hard with your cross-training, it's still a hard day.
5. Never be afraid to take a complete rest day or just take a brisk 30- to 40-minute walk. It may be the best thing for your training.

Part VII

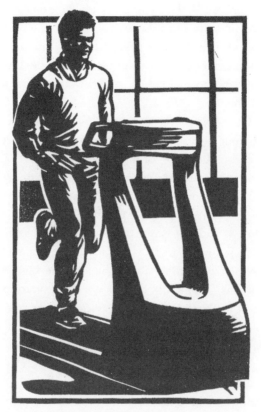

Weight Loss

# Running Works Best

Many runners, both men and women, take up running to lose weight or to maintain a healthy weight. Good reasons. Population studies have shown that the percentage of Americans who are overweight has climbed steadily in the last decade. Up to 20 percent of adults are morbidly obese, and the diagnosis is just as dangerous as it sounds.

Even if the extra pounds spreading around your waist or clinging to your hips don't trigger one of the "lifestyle diseases" like diabetes, heart disease, or high blood pressure, you'll see and feel the pounds. You'll shy away from the mirror, you'll avoid trying on old pants or dresses for another season's wear, and you won't have the energy you'd like to have.

Running is the best way to lose weight and keep it off. To some degree, scientists aren't even sure why. Swimmers can burn as many calories as runners and not lose the same amount of weight. It seems that their bodies want to hold on to some insulation to keep them warm in the water. Bicycling is certainly a good weightloss routine, but you don't hear hundreds of bicycling weight-loss success stories the way you do about running. Walking can work, but often not as quickly and permanently as running.

No matter what your pace, you burn roughly 120 calories per mile of running. The exact number depends on factors such as your current weight and the speed at which you run. At the same time, contrary to popular folklore, running doesn't increase your appetite. It decreases appetite and causes your body to want naturally healthier and more varied food selections.

A very powerful combination. You burn calories but don't get hungry. And when you are ready for the next meal, your body asks you to fill it with nutritious, moderate-fat foods. No wonder running works so well as a weight-loss program.

A little success leads to even greater results. I call this the self-fulfilling cycle of success. Here's what happens. The first miles and pounds are the toughest, of course. But if you stick with a regular, consistent program, you will get through the miles and you will lose a little weight. Since this initial weight loss makes you a more efficient runner, you'll now find it easier to run, which means you'll cover a few more miles. Of course, more miles mean more calories burned, which means more pounds lost, which means you can run easier and farther next week, increasing your calorie burn again.

This doesn't go on endlessly, of course. But once you reach a certain point in your running program—where you can run substantially farther than you could at first—you can actually increase your rate of weight loss. It gets easier and more dramatic, not harder, at least until you reach the healthiest weight for your body. This cycle of success motivates you to stick with the program, guaranteeing that the pounds will steadily come off.

## ❖ Principles ❖

1. Running burns 100 to 140 calories per mile, depending on your weight and pace. This makes it the most efficient calorie-burning activity. You can burn from 300 to 400 calories per half-hour, depending on your individual characteristics. You can easily fit running into your busy lifestyle.
2. Running doesn't increase your appetite. Instead, it makes your body crave a more varied and healthier diet.
3. Because running is what physiologists classify as a vigorous exercise, it revs up your metabolism to the point where your body continues burning calories after you have stopped running. This afterburn can add another 20 percent to your total calorie burn.
4. Running is a four-season activity. You can do it year-round, so you don't fall into an unhealthy yo-yo situation with your weight.
5. You can run anywhere, anytime. You don't need a court or a pool or a tee-off time. You can use a treadmill or open the front door and get in a great calorie-burning workout.

# The Running Diet

To move successfully toward your weight-loss or weight-control goals, you must combine running with sound nutrition. This should be obvious, but it always surprises me how many people think that running gives them the ability to eat anything and everything in sight without worrying about weight gain. It simply doesn't work that way. Yes, there are fat runners!

But not many. Fortunately, running and healthy eating go hand in hand. When you run, your body turns on a sort of feedback loop that asks you to supply it with the nutrients it needs. Instead of turning reflexively to snack foods, fast foods, and other unhealthy food choices, your body begins to crave energy- and nutrient-packed carbohydrates.

The first rule of healthy running and eating is to pay attention to fluids. Runners live and die (literally, though on rare occasions) on fluid balance. You've probably read countless newspaper and magazine stories exhorting you to consume something like eight full glasses of water a day. The articles point out that this is crucial to your health because everything from your blood to your brain requires lots of water for proper high-efficiency functioning.

Well, runners need more than eight glasses, often far more, depending on the amount of daily training they do and the environment they run in. During a race, in fact, physiologists recommend that runners consume as much as six to eight ounces of water or sports drink every 15 to 20 minutes. Of course, you don't need that much when you're sitting around your home or the office, but you get the point: Fluid balance is important.

It also offers you an excellent way to lose or maintain weight while improving your diet. If you begin running more and drinking more water, you'll burn more calories and keep your fluid tank full without consuming more calories. Many runners have used this simple strategy to drop dozens of pounds. It works particularly well when the same individuals had previously been drinking cola, beer, or other calorie-laden beverages.

Despite all the varied and highly promoted diets you hear about every day, sports nutritionists agree that runners should concentrate on carbohydrate-packed foods. That's why so many runners are big consumers of bagels, whole-grain breads, pasta, rice, potatoes, cereals, oatmeal, and energy bars.

For vitamins and minerals, you can't beat vegetables and fruits. Drugstores and health food stores stock a bewildering variety of pills and herbs these days, some of which can provide certain hard-to-get nutrients, but researchers continue to discover that whole foods contain valuable phytochemicals that no pill can package. So eat plenty of the tastiest green, yellow, red, and orange fruits and vegetables you can find.

## ❖ Principles ❖

1. Consume fluids all day long, whether they're water, sports drinks, juices, or soups. Try to take in at least 8 to 10 eight-ounce glasses a day. Consume more when you're running in hot, humid conditions.
2. For maximum weight-loss or weight control, drink water rather than colas and other sweetened beverages. Even fruit juices can be calorie-packed, so drink them in moderation, too.
3. Eat a steady supply of carbohydrates throughout the day to keep your energy at a high level. Bagels are handy and great-tasting, but avoid the cream cheese. Also look for energy bars, which are another good alternative.
4. Avoid high-fat foods, especially snacks and fast foods. When you eat in a hurry, you almost always make unhealthy choices. Give yourself a few more minutes, relax, and eat some real foods.
5. Eat the most richly colorful fruits and vegetables you can find. It turns out that the colors—the greens, yellows, reds, and oranges—indicate an abundance of healthy vitamins and minerals.

# A 24-Hour Program

Running regularly and eating a moderate-calorie, well-balanced diet are the best things you can do for weight loss or healthy weight maintenance. But running—and, indeed, exercise in general—is not the only thing you can do to reach the weight you desire. In fact, when you consider that a five-mile run only burns 500 to 600 calories, you realize that the rest of the day can be more important than your workout time.

Scientists call your daily calorie needs your basic metabolic rate, and you can do much to influence this total, which ranges from 1,800 to 2,800 calories per day in most healthy women and men. Studies have shown, for example, that fidgeters tend to be thinner and healthier than slower, calmer individuals. So one of your health goals should be to develop the habit of fidgeting.

You need not fidget literally, perhaps, but consider where your total daily calorie burn comes from. About 60 to 75 percent comes from your resting metabolic rate (RMR), the number of calories required to maintain necessary body functions. Another 20 to 30 percent comes from your additional daily activities, like cleaning house, walking the supermarket aisles, and exercise. This is your TEA (thermic effect of activity).

A final 5 to 10 percent comes from the energy your body needs to process meals during the day. This is your TEF (thermic effect of feeding). To lose weight, you need to burn more calories through all three channels than you take in. Here are some ways to do this.

Don't go on an overly restrictive diet. When you eat fewer than 1,000 calories a day, your RMR decreases. You don't want this to happen; you want it to increase.

Add strength training to your exercise program. Strength training builds muscle mass, which pumps up your RMR.

Increase your weekly running mileage. The more you run, the more your TEA goes up, and the more calories you burn.

Increase the intensity of your runs. Research has shown that as you run harder, you get more TEA after your workout is completed. This is often called afterburn, and it can add a substantial amount to your total calorie burn.

Eat more often. But make sure that you eat small amounts each time. Studies have shown that you can boost your TEF by eating smaller, more frequent meals during the day. This is called grazing.

Most important, develop the attitude that you're not just exercising to burn more calories. Instead, think about everything you can do to increase your daily metabolic rate. Don't take the elevator; walk up the stairs. Walk the half-mile to the convenience store for that quart of milk. Shovel the snow; don't buy a snowblower.

The best way to get to your healthiest weight is to think of each day as one 24-hour exercise program. Your goal? To get in as many mini-workouts as possible, along with longer exercise periods, like a 30- to 40-minute run.

# ❖ Principles ❖

1. Many studies have shown that exercise holds the key to attaining your best weight. And to use exercise to the maximum, you must think about it in terms of your daily metabolism, or total calorie burn during the day.
2. You can increase your metabolism three ways: more daily activity of all kinds, more traditional exercise, and eating more frequent, smaller meals.
3. Restrictive diets don't work. Rather than boosting your metabolism, they actually slow it down. This is one of many reasons why dieting alone usually isn't effective as a weight-loss program.
4. A strength-training program will help increase your metabolism because muscles burn more calories than other cells. Running more and running faster will also bump up your total calorie burn.
5. Think of every day as a continuous 24-hour exercise program, and get in as many mini-workouts as you can.

# Maximum Weight Loss

While some people run to lose just a few pounds, others have much bigger targets. They want to lose 20, 30, or more pounds. And, naturally, they want the pounds to melt off quickly and easily.

Imagine their surprise—and disgust—when they sometimes gain a pound or two in the first weeks of their training and when their subsequent weight loss is steady but not spectacular.

Running is perhaps the most effective way to lose weight, but that doesn't make it either fast or magical. In fact, you may gain a few pounds early on as your body converts fat tissue to muscle tissue, which is denser and heavier than fat. But if you stick with the program, you'll literally run off the excess pounds.

Here are some of the strategies that have proven most successful for runners interested in maximum weight loss.

Run 25 to 30 miles a week. According to statistics from the National Weight Control Registry, which studies people who have lost at least 30 pounds and kept the weight off, individuals who succeed in their weight-loss efforts burn about 2,800 calories a week through planned exercise. Note that you don't have to run fast or win races, you simply have to be disciplined enough to put in 25 to 30 miles a week of relaxed running.

Run long and slow. Slow workouts that last 90 minutes or more put you into the fat-burning zone, where your body begins to use stored fats, rather than carbohydrates, as a source of fuel. You can't and shouldn't do these longer workouts every day. With good planning, you may be able to fit in two a week. And, yes, it may take you months to work up to a run this long. (For more information, see "Running and Walking" on page 22). Don't be afraid to mix running and walking to reach your goal.

Several times a week, at the end of an easy run, do five or six strides on the grass or on a smooth road surface. Strides are 60- to 80-meter bursts of running at a fast but controlled speed. You don't have to sprint like an Olympian; simply pick up the pace and run smooth and fast for about 10 seconds. Then decelerate, jog for a minute or two until you feel recovered, and do another stride. These bursts of faster running at the end of a workout will boost your afterburn, increasing the number of calories that your body burns after you have finished running.

Eat often and eat everything in moderation. Restrictive diets simply don't work. Everyone falls off the wagon at some point. Better to start the day with a good breakfast, eat many small carbohydrate-packed meals during the day, and even occasionally include small portions of those forbidden, fatty foods. Satisfy your cravings, then get on with your healthy nutrition and exercise program.

# ❖ Principles ❖

1. Running burns more calories than any other simple exercise and has produced more weight-loss success stories than any other activity. But the pounds don't just magically disappear. You must be disciplined and consistent in your training program and take a long-term approach.
2. To lose more weight, run more. You don't have to run fast. You just have to spend the time moving on your feet. The best results seem to come from 25 to 30 miles of running a week.
3. If possible, run 90 minutes or longer several times a week. (Yes, it may take you months to work up to this duration.) Also, do strides several times a week. Both of these strategies can give a boost to your calorie-burning efforts.
4. Drink plenty of water. You can cut up to 15 percent of your daily calorie intake by substituting water for juices, colas, and similar beverages.
5. Don't go on a restrictive very low calorie diet. This will only lower your metabolic rate. Eat breakfast and other carbo-packed meals and snacks regularly throughout the day.

Part VIII

Weather

# Heat

Some world-class runners have been known to joke that they'd like to see the marathon moved from the Summer Olympics to the Winter Olympics. This is their way of saying they'd rather run in cold weather than in hot. And it's true. For runners, heat is much tougher to deal with than cold.

The running body is an intense calorie-burning, heat-producing machine. The heat has to go somewhere. In cool weather, it escapes readily to the air surrounding you. In summer, when that air is 80 to 90°F and perhaps laden with humidity, the heat has no place to go.

You have no place to go, either. You can always dress up for the cold with more or better clothing, but how do you dress down for the heat? You can only go so far.

Instead, you have to accommodate the conditions. You have to adjust the way you normally run, to be sure that you don't become overheated and dehydrated. Otherwise, you risk suffering from some degree of heat illness, which can range from the unpleasant (dizziness or nausea) to the downright deadly.

Most of the steps you should take are simple common sense. First, don't run during the heat of the day. Look for the long shadows of early morning or late afternoon. Or seek out places, like forest trails or waterfront runs, that provide relief from the sun and the most intense heat.

Second, run less and run slower. Most heat-illness cases among runners strike those who are extremely motivated to achieve something. Usually, that something is a race goal. Trust me, you're not going to set any records when racing in the heat. So relax, lower your expectations, and run slower. Don't be concerned about your time. As soon as the weather turns cool again, you can return to faster running.

Summer can be a tough time to train for a marathon. If

you're aiming for a fall marathon, save your hardest long runs until after Labor Day, when you may get some breaks in the weather. Or get them done early in the morning, before the worst summer heat settles in. The best advice of all is to run long workouts with a friendly, helpful group in which everyone takes care of everyone else and makes a point of stopping frequently for fluids and energy snacks.

Runners usually have the most trouble with heat during the first steamy week of summer. Their bodies haven't adapted yet, and the sudden heat and humidity jolt their systems hard. Don't push yourself at times like this. Give yourself several weeks to get accustomed to the summer conditions. Your body has marvelous adaptation abilities. Just give them a chance to kick in. You'll never run as easily or as fast in summer as you do in spring or fall, but you can run comfortably and safely.

# ❖ Principles ❖

1. Drink, drink, drink in the hours leading up to your run, especially in the 15 minutes before you run. Keep rehydrating during your run. You get the message—drink.
2. Run at the coolest times of the day or in the coolest places. Early mornings and late afternoons are best. Forested parks can provide relief from the heat, as can running courses near lakes and the seashore.
3. Run less and run slower than at other times of the year. Don't expect to set any records in races.
4. If you begin to feel dizzy or nauseated, stop running and get into the shade. Have someone bring you water for drinking and to soak your body. Do the same for your friends and training partners. In the summer, runners have to watch out for and take care of each other.
5. Give yourself time to adapt to hot weather. It can take several weeks. During this period, run regularly, but don't run hard.

# Cold

In summer, sweating is your body's natural way of trying to cool itself down. In winter, though, sweat can be a bad thing. When you sweat on a cold day, the water evaporates, chilling your body and possibly leading to hypothermia.

During the summer, of course, there's nothing you can do about sweating. It only becomes a problem when you exercise too hard or too long without maintaining your fluid balance. Stop sweating in the heat, and you're in trouble.

In winter, you can do something about sweating. Dress only as warmly as necessary to keep yourself dry and comfortable. Don't dress so warmly that you start sweating a lot. Overdressing in cold weather is the mistake of an inexperienced runner and is more likely to leave you cold and chilled than wearing lighter clothes is.

For some reason, it took me years to comprehend this simple lesson. Thirty years ago, I tried to beat the cold by bundling up in several layers of thick cotton sweatshirts. After 10 minutes of moderate running, I'd be sweating nicely and congratulating myself for dealing with the elements. Another 20 to 30 minutes later, however, I would change direction slightly on my workout, and suddenly feel the wind. It would pierce through my clothing, evaporate the sweat on my body, and leave me chilled and uncomfortable even as I continued running.

Eventually, I got the message. If I didn't dress so heavily on these runs, I wouldn't sweat as much and wouldn't get so cold. I wore less clothing, felt a tad exposed for the first five minutes of a run, and then reached a comfort zone as my body warmed up. The rest of my workout was perfect.

At about the same time, the clothing produced for running and other vigorous outdoor activities improved dramatically. Apparel scientists realized that runners needed shirts, sweatshirts, and shells that moved sweat away from the body—which cotton doesn't do—and also blocked the wind from penetrating. Today, we have a wide variety of microfiber garments to choose from, and they perform as nothing before them ever has.

As a result, you can control your own microenvironment in the apparel surrounding your body. With a microfiber hat on your head and a zipped-up microfiber windjacket, you're ready to tackle the windy portions of your workout route. When you turn and have the wind at your back, take off your hat and unzip the jacket halfway to make sure that you don't start sweating too much. Control is the key concept. Dress in a flexible manner that lets you adjust options as the wind and temperature change.

If winter forces you to sometimes run in the dark, be sure to wear various reflective apparel, and make visibility your top priority.

## ❖ Principles ❖

1. Don't overdress. Strive for a balanced approach that will keep you warm but not so warm that you start sweating a lot.
2. Protect the extremities first—hands, ears, nose, and, for men, the genital area. The extremities are the most exposed to cold and wind and the most susceptible to frostbite.
3. Buy breathable, microfiber clothing for winter runs. The t-shirt will wick sweat away from your body. A microfiber shell—buy one with a full zipper—will continue doing the same and should also have some wind-blocking properties. In extremely cold conditions, you may need a breathable, insulating layer between your shirt and shell.
4. Dress flexibly for conditions that change as you run. Put on your hat and zip up your jacket when running into a cold wind. Take the hat off and zip the jacket down halfway when running with the wind at your back.
5. Don't worry too much about your legs and feet. Your legs need much less protection than your torso needs, and few runners complain of cold feet. Their feet are just too busy to get cold.

# Dark, Snow, Ice, and Rain

Weather conditions can bring a variety of challenges as well as spectacular beauty to your running. Most runners leap at the opportunity to log a few easy miles on a sparkling cold mid-winter's night just after a soft, crunchy snow has fallen. And no workout can match the freshness of a trail run in a soft, mild summer rainfall.

That said, these and other weather conditions also cause many workouts to be canceled and sometimes introduce safety concerns. Darkness is the most dangerous, both because you are less visible to passing vehicles and because you can't see the ground.

Safety is the overriding concern, and the first rule is to accept responsibility for protecting yourself. In the dark, you must pay particular attention to vehicle traffic, and always run with extreme caution. Remember to run on the left side of the road, facing traffic, so you can see oncoming vehicles.

To make sure car drivers see you, wear reflective gear on your torso and some moving part of your body—the movement is what catches the driver's eye. Many runner's jackets, pants, and even shoes have reflective strips. You can also buy reflective vests and reflective Velcro bands that wrap around your arms or lower legs. Find something—or even better, several things—that is comfortable enough that you'll wear it everytime you run in the dark.

To avoid falls, sprained ankles, and the like, run on smooth roads with wide shoulders. Once you've found a course or two that works well for your routine, stick with it. Carry a small flashlight to illuminate any unusual objects, and run at a slow, comfortable pace to avoid stumbles. Darkness doesn't lend itself to hard, fast running, so don't get tempted. If you must do some hard training in the dark, find a lightly traveled hill and run hill repeats.

Snow and ice can make the footing treacherous, leading to falls and accidents. Black ice poses obvious dangers to both runners and cars and makes it dangerous to be sharing the road. The trickiest time of day is often dusk, when the roads are full of vehicles, darkness is settling, and snow or water is freezing. Be particularly cautious when running at this time.

Rain is a threat mainly because of the way it can obscure both your visibility and a driver's. In a pelting rain, you may be looking down (to protect your eyes) rather than up, and a driver will have trouble peering through his windshield wipers. If a rain turns cold and windy, it can also lead to a rapid drop in your body temperature, so it's a good idea to run roads close to home if you suspect such conditions. Water-resistant or waterproof gear can help, but there are no guarantees in a hard, lashing rain.

# ❖ Principles ❖

1. When running in the dark, wear reflective gear at all times. A reflective vest is good, and additional reflective material on your arms and lower legs is even better.
2. Always remember that car drivers can't see you as well as you can see them. Run on the left side of the road, facing traffic, and give a wide berth to passing traffic. Run slowly and conservatively, without any sudden bursts of speed or attempts to cross over to the other side of the road.
3. Run on well-maintained roads that have wide, smooth shoulders. Carry a small flashlight to illuminate any unusual objects.
4. Remember that any weather that makes conditions more dangerous for cars makes things much more dangerous for you. When running in rain, snow, or ice, you must be especially alert and cautious.
5. Don't tempt fate by trying to run hard and fast in the dark or in other difficult weather. If you must do a hard workout, run repeats on a lightly trafficked hill or run on an indoor track.

# Part IX

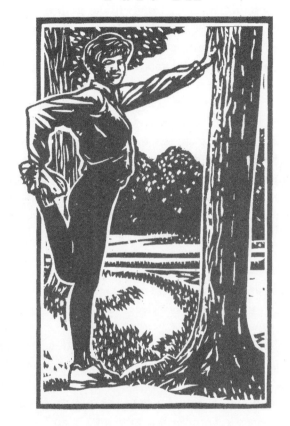

# Injury Prevention and Treatment

# Overuse Injuries

Some people simply can't run without getting injured (because they have severe structural problems), and some can go almost forever without getting hurt. But most runners are right in the middle. They can run and improve their health and racing, but they're also susceptible to injuries when not careful.

The most common cause of injuries in runners is overuse syndrome. This is often described as doing too much, too fast, too soon. It strikes beginning runners, to be sure, but it can also surprise veteran runners who suddenly decide to increase their training, thinking that they're too experienced and too smart to get injured.

To avoid overuse syndrome, first follow the 10-percent rule (for more information, see page 20). Make sure that you increase your training mileage in a slow, consistent manner. Follow the same rule with your long runs.

Also, be careful with speedwork and hills. Running fast puts your body in an entirely different position (leaning forward, up on your forefeet) that can stress the feet, Achilles tendons, and knees more than slower running.

When you start a speedwork program, be careful not to run at your top speed the first week. Gradually ease into your speed sessions. The first week, do relatively little running at a relatively moderate pace, and each subsequent week, run more and faster. In other words, give your body time to adapt.

Do the same with hill training. In some ways, running up hills can be less stressful than flat running, because you produce less impact force. But it also puts your body in a different position, which creates new and different forces. Be careful about downhill running, because it increases impact forces several fold.

You also need to change your training shoes regularly to prevent overuse injuries. The midsoles, the most important parts of training shoes, lose much of their cushioning and stability after

300 to 500 miles. If you continue to run on worn midsoles, you may suffer injuries due to both impact forces and overpronation, which is excessive inward rolling of the foot when landing.

If possible, buy two pairs of shoes at once, and alternate them between workouts. Presumably, they will put your feet in slightly different positions. This way, you won't repeat the same pattern in the same shoes day after day—the very definition of overuse syndrome.

Most important of all, take time off at the first sign of an injury. Skip three days to see if that helps. Try walking instead of running, or use the pool or stationary bike. Then try a short run. If the injury feels better, gradually return to your old routine.

If this doesn't work, take a week off and try again while treating yourself with ice and anti-inflammatories. Still no success? It's time to consider seeing a doctor. Ask around and find a sports-medicine specialist rather than a general practitioner. You want a doctor who understands why running is important to you.

## ❖ Principles ❖

1. Overuse injuries happen to most runners. Fortunately, the vast majority are soft-tissue injuries that spontaneously heal themselves in 3 to 10 days. Don't run on these injuries. Use rest, ice, and anti-inflammatories, and give them the chance to heal.

2. To prevent overuse injuries, always run less and slower than you think you should. Avoid the too much, too fast, too soon trap. Even Olympic champions run slowly and comfortably most days of the week.

3. When you increase your training mileage, add no more than 10 percent per week. Boost your workouts more than that, and you're asking for trouble.

4. Be particularly careful about speedwork and hills. Both can provoke injuries and require a gradual adaptation process.

5. Be sure to buy training shoes every 300 to 500 miles. If possible, buy two pairs and alternate them between workouts.

# Stretching

Runners have always been told to stretch to prevent injuries. And they always will be told to stretch, I believe. Although, in truth, no large, well-controlled study has ever shown stretching to be effective in preventing injuries.

It's the airtight theory behind stretching that convinces us of its effectiveness. Running produces stronger but tighter muscles, particularly at the back of the body—the calves, hamstrings, and back muscles. And runners get injuries, often in these same muscle groups. So it makes sense that gentle stretching should help alleviate some of the muscle tightness and resulting injuries.

The key word is "gentle." Harsh, fast, ballistic stretching is more likely to cause problems than to prevent them. The yoga approach—slow, quiet, peaceful—works much better. In fact, many runners practice yoga as their preferred form of stretching.

Over the years, many other forms of stretching have been developed. Some use towels and cords, some require partners, some involve long sequences of dozens of specific positions. Given how little is known about stretching's effectiveness, I certainly can't say that one of these systems is better or worse than another.

But I can say this: Go slowly, and don't stretch past the point of pain. The idea is simply to reach the point where you feel a slight tightness in the muscle group, and then to relax for 20 to 30 seconds at that point. Repeat the stretch 6 to 10 times, each time striving only for complete relaxation. Regular stretching of this type should gradually increase the muscle's range of motion, making you more flexible and more resistant to injuries.

Stretching should be performed when the muscle group is warm, not cold. That makes evening a better time than morning and after your workout a better time than before. It's best to warm up by easing into a run very gradually, and then to include 5 to 15 minutes of stretching in the post-run cooldown.

As I mentioned, you can find dozens of different stretching positions in books and magazines. But nobody has time for all of them. So let's go straight to the two best stretches for runners.

***Achilles-calf stretch.*** Often called the wall pushup, this exercise stretches the calf muscle, taking pressure off the Achilles tendon. Stand several feet from a wall with one leg in front of the other, both pointing straight ahead, and place your palms on the wall. While keeping your rear leg straight, with your heel firmly planted on the ground, bend your front knee and lean into the wall as far as possible (without pain). Hold for 20 seconds, repeat nine more times, and switch legs.

***Hamstring stretch.*** Straighten one leg and place that foot on a chair. Bend forward over that leg, reaching your hands toward your foot. Stop when you feel a tension in your hamstring. Hold for 20 seconds, repeat nine more times, and switch legs.

# ❖ Principles ❖

1. Although unproven by any conclusive research studies, stretching makes sense as an injury-prevention method. Since it lengthens and relaxes the muscles that are made shorter and stronger by running, it should make these same muscles less "brittle" and more injury-resistant.
2. Stretch slowly and gradually. Don't stretch beyond the point of pain. Consider yoga as an effective stretching program.
3. Hold each stretch for 20 to 30 seconds, uncoil slowly, and repeat 6 to 10 times. Use towels, a rope, a partner, or whatever system works for you. Just be sure to keep it slow and gentle.
4. Stretch after you are warmed up, not before. Stretch at the end of a workout or race. Five to 15 minutes of gentle stretching will help you recover for your next workout.
5. Concentrate on your calf muscles and your hamstrings. Stretching these muscles will provide the greatest injury-prevention payoff for most runners.

# Ice

Ice is often the simplest, fastest, and most effective means of preventing and treating an injury. The moment you notice the kind of slightly inflamed soreness that indicates the first stage of a soft-tissue injury, you should turn to ice. Similarly, when you have an acute or chronic injury, ice can play a major role in your recovery and return to pain-free running.

Ice works by limiting the inflammation at the injured tissue. A little inflammation is good; indeed, it's essential to the healing process. But too much produces pain, limits your range of motion in the injured area, and retards your return to full health.

You've probably heard reference to RICE as an injury-fighting treatment. RICE refers to rest, ice, compression, and elevation. All are self-explanatory, and the first two are by far the most important. Rest prevents further injury to the problem area, and ice promotes the actual recovery of the injured tissues.

The sooner you can apply the ice, the better, which is why you should always have one or several forms of ice at the ready in your freezer. The form of ice you choose doesn't make a huge difference. But having it there does.

Traditionally, athletic trainers kept themselves surrounded by ice cubes and various kinds of bags, ranging from rubber to plastic. When an injured athlete needed ice, the trainer simply popped some cubes into a bag and placed the bag on the inflamed body part. You can do the same at home.

Of course, you have many other alternatives. One is the flexible ice pack, available in most drugstores, that contains a gel that remains flexible when frozen. This allows you to actually wrap the ice pack around your body. In fact, with one of these packs, you can apply ice and compression at the same time.

Even simpler and just about as handy is a small bag of frozen peas or corn. The frozen veggie pack has a modest degree of flexibility, and you can wrap it around your injury with a cloth or towel.

Finally, many runners put several paper cups full of water in the freezer and use the resulting ice cup for direct application and massage to an injured muscle. As the ice melts and gets smaller, you can tear off a little paper from the lip of the cup to reveal more ice for the next application.

Whichever form of ice you choose, follow this procedure: (1) apply the ice to the injury as soon as possible; (2) leave the ice on for only 10 to 15 minutes at a time to avoid frostbite; (3) repeat the icing several times a day; (4) continue icing until the injury and inflammation are completely gone; (5) return to running very slowly and conservatively; (6) continue the icing process after each workout until you feel certain the injury has healed completely.

## ❖ Principles ❖

1. By quickly applying ice to areas of soreness and inflammation, you can often prevent them from developing into more serious injuries. Similarly, ice should be the first line of defense against an acute injury like an ankle sprain.
2. Follow the RICE advice. In addition to ice, you must use rest in battling injury. Compression and elevation are also helpful, but less essential.
3. Always keep ice in the freezer and train yourself to use it frequently. All forms are good, including ice cubes, frozen gel packs, frozen vegetables, and cups of frozen water.
4. Apply ice as many times a day as you can, but only for 10 to 15 minutes at a time. More than that, and you risk frostbite to the skin.
5. When the injury and inflammation are gone, return very slowly and gradually to your training program. Continue to use ice after your workouts. To use ice is to follow the age-old wisdom "An ounce of prevention is worth a pound of cure."

# Pain Relievers

When you feel some inevitable aches and pains the day after a hard workout, it's tempting to pop the first painkilling medication you can put your hands on. You'll be even more tempted if you're in the middle of a marathon training program or getting ready for a big race. But should you use the painkillers? Sometimes, yes; but not all the time.

The problem with painkillers is that some runners get nearly addicted to them. The pills are not physically addictive, but the ease with which they mask pain make them attractive. Like all strong medicines, they have potentially harmful side effects.

Of the leading painkillers, aspirin, ibuprofen, naproxen sodium, and ketoprofen are also anti-inflammatories. This makes them particularly attractive to runners, who are always looking for ways to reduce muscle inflammation. Acetaminophen is a painkiller but not an anti-inflammatory.

The major drawback to all the anti-inflammatories is that they can also produce stomach irritation. If you take too many anti-inflammatories for too long, you may develop gastric bleeding and ulcers. There's also some evidence that taking anti-inflammatories during a very hot workout or a marathon can reduce blood flow to the kidneys, a potentially dangerous condition. The Food and Drug Administration has begun to approve a new group of prescription anti-inflammatories that don't produce stomach irritation. You may want to ask your doctor about these new drugs.

It's not the potentially harmful side effects that bother me the most, though. It's runners who use the medicines to mask pain, rather than resolving the root cause. I'd rather see you using rest, cross-training, ice, stretching, and strengthening to cure an injury and prevent it from reoccurring.

That said, you can use an over-the-counter anti-inflammatory as part of a short-term program for injury recovery. Use the following program for 10 days, then stop. If your injury is not completely healed, see a doctor. Do not return to using the anti-inflammatory.

Take three anti-inflammatory pills four times a day. This is 50 percent more than the recommended dosage but less than a doctor would prescribe for you on a short-term basis. Take plenty of fluids with each dose of the pills.

While on this program, rest the injured muscle group. Also, ice it as much as possible. You can cross-train if that doesn't tax the injury. Remember, you're only sticking to this regimen for 10 days, so you may as well do everything you can to make it successful.

After 10 days, stop taking the medication, and return very gradually to your running. Don't go far and don't go fast. With luck, you'll be able to build back to your desired level of training, and the injury won't reoccur.

# ❖ Principles ❖

1. Over-the-counter (OTC) painkillers should only be used for short-term relief of running-induced muscle aches and pains. They should not become an everyday crutch or a mask for injuries.
2. Many of the OTC painkillers are also anti-inflammatories (acetaminophen is the exception). These can help reduce muscle inflammation, but they can also produce gastric irritation.
3. Don't take anti-inflammatories before or during long, hard runs or marathons. The anti-inflammatories tend to reduce blood flow to the kidneys. When combined with dehydration, this can produce a dangerous condition.
4. For short-term, at-home recovery from a muscle injury, take three over-the-counter anti-inflammatory pills four times a day for 10 days. Don't run; do ice the injury as much as possible.
5. If the injury is cured by this procedure, return very gradually to your training. If it's not, consult a sports-medicine doctor. Do not continue taking the anti-inflammatory.

# Shinsplints

Shinsplints are possibly the most common injury faced by beginning runners and, fortunately, are one of the easiest to recover from. Generally, shinsplints—pain and soreness along the fronts of the lower legs—affect leg muscles that are not yet accustomed to the rigors of running. As a result, beginners are particularly susceptible, as are veterans returning to a program or anyone who suddenly switches his training or training surface.

The best immediate treatment for shinsplints is rest, combined with icing and anti-inflammatories. Ice the area for 10 to 15 minutes after running as well as several other times a day. Also, begin taking an anti-inflammatory like aspirin or ibuprofen, and continue taking it on a regular schedule for 10 days. If possible, try the compression (taping) and elevation that make up the other two parts of the RICE prescription.

If your shinsplints are moderate, you may be able to run through them without taking a complete rest. Instead, decrease your training by 30 to 50 percent, stick to only slow running on the flats, and switch from hard surfaces like concrete to smooth, firm grass and dirt surfaces. Lastly, follow the ice and anti-inflammatory regimen. If this doesn't prove effective after a week or so, take a complete break from your running and substitute other forms of cross-training that don't stress your lower legs.

You can help your shin muscles grow stronger with a simple exercise. Sit on the edge of a table. Loop a light weight—many runners use a bag filled with sand—over one foot at a time, and lift the weight by flexing only your ankle. Don't bend your knee.

You can perform a similar shin-strengthening exercise with an elastic band or tension tubing that is increasingly available at drugstores and sporting goods stores. Tie one end of the band to a heavy object such as a table leg and loop the other end around the forefoot of your injured foot. Sit facing the heavy object and flex your foot toward you and side to side against the band's resistance. Again, use your ankle, not your knee.

A new pair of shoes can also be helpful in relieving shinsplints. First, the new shoes may provide increased shock absorption. Second, you can buy motion-control shoes to keep your feet from overpronating and placing additional twisting forces on your shin muscles from the excessive inward rolling of your feet when they land. If your shinsplints prove unusually painful and hard to get rid of, consult a sports-medicine podiatrist to see if you need orthotics.

When running through shinsplints or returning to running after shinsplints, always stick to flat, smooth, soft surfaces. Avoid rough, uneven surfaces, as they will torque your feet and shins. Practice good form; don't lean forward, don't overstride, and don't land on your toes unless that is natural to you.

# ❖ Principles ❖

1. Shinsplints are common, particularly among beginning runners, but not serious; and they are easy to treat. At the first sign of shinsplint pain, begin icing the irritated area and taking anti-inflammatories. Continue this regimen for 10 days.
2. If necessary, rest or cross-train for several weeks to relieve stress to the lower legs. Buy a new pair of shoes with greater cushioning and motion control.
3. Strengthen your shin muscles with foot-leg exercises that force you to work against resistance by flexing your ankles only. Don't bend your knees, as this will engage other muscle groups.
4. When you return to running, avoid hills, speedwork, and hard surfaces. Try to find a grassy area or dirt road with a smooth, even surface. Don't run on uneven surfaces, even soft ones.
5. Practice good running form. Don't lean forward, don't overstride, and don't land on your toes or forefeet (unless this is natural for you). Run with a comfortable, erect body carriage—head over shoulders over hips over heels.

# Knee Injuries

In almost every study of injured runners, knee injuries have topped the list of complaints. In many cases, the injuries begin with football, basketball, tennis, or skiing accidents and return many years later in running programs. And if you are a big runner with flat feet, you have more of a tendency to overpronate, which can cause knee problems. Pronation is the natural inward turning of the foot as it lands and rolls through the heel-to-toe movement of a running stride.

At the first sign of an aching knee, take several days off, begin a course of anti-inflammatories, and ice all around the knee joint three or four times a day. If you get relief, return to walking and then running on a very gradual basis, and avoid hills (especially downhills) until you feel that your knee is at full strength again.

Some knee injuries—those that are caused by mild overpronation—can be resolved by a change of shoes. Because overpronation is so common, every major shoe company makes several shoes specifically for this problem. These are generally called motion-control shoes. You will recognize motion-control shoes because they're beefier than other shoes, with more plastic and hard-rubber devices on the inside edges of the shoes to limit pronation.

Leg-strengthening exercises can also help prevent future knee pain. The quadriceps muscles on the fronts of your thighs maintain your knees in their proper alignments, so quadriceps-strengthening routines will help your knees. At the same time, you should do strengthening exercises and flexibility stretches for your hamstrings, the opposing muscle groups at the backs of your thighs.

When all else fails, many runners find that they can obtain knee relief from orthotics, custom-fitted foot appliances that are prescribed, fitted, and ordered by a sports podiatrist. Find a podiatrist who understands the biomechanics of running, and have him perform a gait analysis of your running form as well as a physical check on your feet and legs. Orthotics can control overpronation, leg-length discrepancies, and other conditions that may be limiting your running pleasure.

When you return to running, make sure you don't do too much, too soon. Build your training gradually and avoid downhill running. Be prepared for adjustments to your training program.

For example, some runners with knee pain have to be sure to always take a day off between running workouts. Others quickly learn exactly how much running their knees can absorb in a week without breaking down—it may be 15 miles, 30 miles, or 50 miles. Once you find what works for you, don't cheat. You'll be far happier if you keep your knees healthy.

## ❖ Principles ❖

1. Though often caused by prior injuries, knee pain is the most common runners' injury. If your knee begins to ache, stop running for several days and treat with anti-inflammatories and ice.
2. Begin a quadriceps-strengthening program. The quadriceps muscle groups, just above your knees, are responsible for holding your knees in their proper alignments.
3. Also, consider a new pair of shoes. Knee pain is often caused by overpronation, which is particularly common among heavier runners with low arches or flat feet. Motion-control shoes can help limit overpronation.
4. You may need custom orthotics, fitted by a sports podiatrist. Orthotics provide custom, balanced foundations for your feet, legs, and running stride.
5. When returning to running after a knee injury, proceed with particular care. Build your mileage very gradually. Use ice and anti-inflammatories after workouts. Avoid downhill running, which greatly magnifies the impact forces of running. Recognize that you may have to take rest days after your running days and limit your weekly mileage.

# Achilles Tendinitis

The Achilles is a heroic tendon at the back of the heel that's responsible for bearing the full weight of the body with each running stride. Unfortunately, this means that the Achilles tendon must absorb tremendous stress, and as a result, it occasionally suffers an injury.

Often, this injury occurs when you make a dramatic change in your training. For example, you increase your mileage abruptly or enter several races in rapid succession.

Either of these could trigger Achilles inflammation, more commonly known as tendinitis, or the rarer, and more serious, Achilles rupture. To prevent Achilles problems, follow the golden rule of training: Increase your mileage gradually, no more than 10 percent per week, and avoid sudden changes in your program.

You should begin treating an Achilles tendon injury as soon as you notice the first soreness and tightness in the Achilles area behind your ankle. Begin by taking several days off from running and icing the tendon for 15 to 20 minutes three or four times a day.

You can also take painkilling anti-inflammatories like aspirin or ibuprofen to reduce the swelling that's causing the tendon stiffness. It's generally quite safe to take 50 percent more anti-inflammatory than the label recommends. This is still less than a doctor would likely give you as a prescription anti-inflammatory, and the additional dosage will greatly enhance the anti-inflammatory effect.

Closely follow the directions to take the painkiller four times a day so that your bloodstream has a sufficiently high level of anti-inflammatory around the clock. Stop after 10 days.

You can also put slight heel lifts in your dress shoes to prevent your Achilles from overextending during everyday walking. When you return to running, put the heel lifts in your running shoes.

You don't want to start a stretching program while your Achilles is acting up, but you'll certainly want to begin stretching as soon as your Achilles gets better. Concentrate on stretching exercises for the calf muscles (the soleus and gastrocnemius), as tight calf muscles often contribute to Achilles problems.

If your Achilles has been injured for some time and has developed scar tissue, you may consider having a physical therapist or massage therapist try several sessions of cross-fiber friction massage. This technique is the opposite of the relaxing massage everyone loves. It hurts because the therapist uses forceful, probing movements to break up the scarring that has developed around your Achilles. If successful, this technique can provide significant relief.

When you run again, be sure to select shoes that have firm, stable bases of support in the rear feet and good forefeet flexibility so your Achilles won't have to work too hard at toeoff, the part of your stride when you push off with your foot.

## ❖ Principles ❖

1. At the first sign of Achilles tendinitis, take several days off from running and begin icing the tendon. Ice the Achilles three or four times a day for 15 to 20 minutes each time.
2. You can also use painkilling anti-inflammatories like aspirin or ibuprofen to limit the swelling and inflammation around the Achilles. Be sure to follow directions and take the anti-inflammatory around the clock to guarantee that a sufficient amount remains in your bloodstream all the time.
3. Don't stretch while your Achilles is still sore, but begin a regular calf stretching program after you move beyond the initial injury stage. Also, put small heel lifts in your dress shoes and running shoes to limit the overextension of your Achilles.
4. Consider getting several cross-fiber friction massages from a physical therapist or massage therapist. While briefly painful, this sort of forceful massage can prove very effective.
5. When you return to running, select shoes with firm, stable bases of support in the rear feet and good flexibility in the forefeet.

# Part X

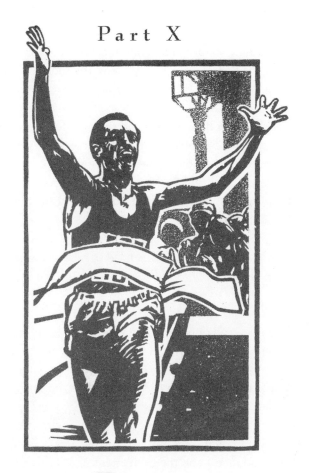

# Racing

# The Decision to Race

Most runners follow a fairly predictable pattern of racing frequently in their early years. They enjoy the "burn" of racing and the chance to improve their times, which lasts, on average, about seven years.

After that, you hit a plateau and then gradually slow down as you get older. You'll probably enter fewer races and begin to concentrate more on the other benefits of running—the stress relief, the vitality, the healthfulness of it. If you don't have a shot at any age-group awards, you may find yourself asking the question, "Why should I race?"

It's an important question for runners of all ages and one that deserves close scrutiny. You don't need to race to lower your cholesterol level or for enhanced weight control, and you certainly don't need to race to control your high blood pressure. Why, then, should you race?

The answer can only come from you and your personal needs. I have heard many highly paid executives tell me that their daily lives are so frenzied and competitive that the last thing they need in life is another hurry-up race. They use their running to get away from it all. A perfectly good reason to run.

At the same time, I know other people who feel that they don't receive enough recognition in their lives. They crave an arena—a road race—and the excitement of a starting line. These people never feel so fully alive as when they are chasing down other runners in a race, listening to the roar of the crowd, waiting for the triumphant moment when they cross the finish line with their arms raised in the air.

Most runners fall in between these two extremes, and that's why we enter races. Sometimes, we feel like joining thousands of others as we take over the streets in a fast-paced and colorful parade, or we feel like testing ourselves to see what we can produce, or we feel that a race is a celebration of ourselves, our friends, and our shared passion for running.

As a result, we race whenever the spirit moves us. We are thankful for the thousands of weekend races across the country, even when we don't always feel like entering them, because we like the idea of choice. If we didn't have so many opportunities, we might feel compelled to look harder for races.

Simply knowing that the races are there gives us comfort. It gives us a chance to race in the places and at the distances we select. Choosing one's own path, whether on a daily workout or for a weekend race, lies at the very heart of running. It gives us the freedom we crave.

## ❖ Principles ❖

1. Some runners should race, some shouldn't. Only you can decide how racing may affect you. Whatever you choose, stay flexible, and feel free to change your mind. Remember, runners do not have to race.
2. The motivation struggle lies at the heart of any exercise program, and races can be great motivators. Use them to keep motivated and excited about your running. And don't just aim for fast times. Reward yourself by taking a trip to a race you've always wanted to enter.
3. The occasional race can be an important part of a training program. When using races as part of a plan geared toward a big, season-ending event, you generally shouldn't race more than once every two weeks.
4. Don't overrace. Racing too often is one of the most common causes of overtraining and staleness.
5. Make races playful, social situations. Don't be afraid to run a race for fun, and don't worry about time. Just enjoy the opportunity to join your friends, see a new city, or run through scenic trails.

# Goals

Once you've decided to enter a race, a question pops up: What's your goal? Or, what are your expectations for this race? This question looks innocent enough, but it can have a major impact on your future running and racing.

Goals have good and bad sides, in running and in life. They give you something concrete to aim for, keep you focused, and provide a good reason for celebration after the race if everything goes as planned. But goals can also focus too much on performance rather than on enjoyment, can become all-consuming, and can leave you feeling disappointed if you fail to achieve them.

To avoid this, always emphasize the positive aspects of goal setting over the negative. You do this by setting realistic goals.

The best way is to establish at least three different goals for any race. Say you're entering your first marathon. You know it would be silly to aim too high. After all, the marathon is going to be difficult enough without adding an unattainable time.

Instead, set three levels of performance goals—one quite easy to attain, one moderately difficult, and the third representing a dream-but-doable goal. For a first-time marathoner with little racing experience, these three goals might be (1) to finish the race, (2) to finish in under 5 hours, (3) to finish in under 4½ hours.

Some runners find it difficult to set less-than-Olympian goals like these, because they feel that they're being too wimpy. Take another look, however, and you'll realize that this isn't the case. Unless you are a runner of Olympic potential, merely finishing your first marathon does represent a great accomplishment.

After all, what percentage of the population has run a marathon? Maybe one-tenth of 1 percent? That by itself practically makes you a superstar.

Besides, even Olympians don't usually break records in their first marathons. They, too, begin with realistic goals. They know it will take years for them to hone their skills. Just because you don't aim particularly high in your first marathon doesn't mean that you can't raise the bar in subsequent efforts.

In establishing goals, don't forget that there are hundreds of important reasons for racing in addition to the final time on the race clock. You can have health goals, charity fund-raising goals, running-a-race-in-every-state goals, and so on.

Don't let traditional thinking limit your options. You own your racing experience, so you don't have to rely on other people's expectations. You can turn your race, and your goals for the race, into anything you want.

And the best thing you can possibly do is to make the race fun and motivating. That way you'll want to keep running and racing.

## ❖ Principles ❖

1. The number one reason for setting race goals is to increase your motivation and focus. The goal of goal setting, you might say, is to produce a positive outcome.
2. To increase the likelihood of a positive outcome, set goals that are attainable. Establishing impossible-dream goals is too likely to disappoint and depress you.
3. To make sure you achieve your performance goals, give yourself a range of goals, including a very attainable goal, a slightly more difficult goal, and a dream-but-doable goal.
4. Remember that performance goals are just a tiny part of a much bigger picture. Also, set goals that are more personal and more experiential. Again, keep them doable. And reward yourself when you achieve them.
5. As soon as you have finished one race and achieved one set of goals, set your sights on a different event that requires a different set of goals. Pick something that will be both fun and involving. Another goal of goal setting is to keep you motivated by continually introducing new challenges.

# Mental Preparation

After they decide to enter a race, most runners spend weeks, if not months, training for that race. They tailor their schedules to include certain key workouts that get them in peak condition, they watch what they eat more carefully than usual, and they spend more time on stretching and other injury-prevention activities.

But they often don't pay enough attention to the mental side of their preparation, which is probably more important than all the others combined. You can make sure you have this base covered by following a mental program that begins well in advance of your big race and contains strategies to use during the actual competition.

There are many small ways to do this. Separately, they may not seem to amount to much, but together they can make a significant contribution toward helping you run your best. They will guarantee that you don't waste all those good training miles on a race where you get mentally sidetracked and don't achieve your goals.

To begin, set aside a few minutes every day to visualize yourself running the race. (A good time to do this is when you've finished showering after a workout.) Close your eyes and imagine the nervousness you'll feel beforehand, the thrill of the start, the middle miles, and the drive to the finish. In each of these scenarios, picture yourself remaining calm and in control, running smooth and relaxed.

Okay, no race is easy, and nothing ever goes perfectly. Let's say you hit some tough hills in the last third of the race. No fun. Hills are always difficult, and you're already tired. You're obviously not going to prance up these hills like a gazelle in the wilds.

But if you've done your visualization homework, you'll cope just fine. You're not going to collapse, and you won't have to start walking. You know you'll soon reach the top of the hill, and then things will get better.

When the going gets really hard—and we all know that happens—here are several additional tactics. Break the rest of the race into small pieces, miles, or even quarter-miles. Things are always easier when you concentrate on just one small task at a time.

Acknowledge the fatigue and pain you're feeling. Talk to your discomfort, and I mean this quite literally, silly as it sounds. When you have a conversation with your fatigue, you demystify it, taking away much of its power and control over you.

Make a bargain with your body. Tell it that if it will just cooperate and get you to the finish, you'll treat it really nicely afterward. Maybe you'll give it a hot bath or cover it with nice-smelling oils or reward it with a massage. For sure, you won't make it do something this hard again until it's fully recovered.

# ❖ Principles ❖

1. Having a mental-preparation plan for your races is as important as having a training schedule. More bad races result from little or no mental preparation than from poor training.
2. Use visualization techniques (mental pictures) before the race to imagine yourself running a smooth, controlled effort. Stay calm. Don't panic over anything that happens. You can cope.
3. On race day, continuing using these mental pictures to get you through the tough spots. Missed a water stop? That's okay. You'll survive if you just keep running relaxed until you reach the next one.
4. In the second half of the race, as the pain and fatigue grow, break the race into small sections and attack just one at a time. You don't have three miles to go to the 10-K finish line. You only have one mile to go until you reach the next mile marker.
5. Toward the end, shift your attention inward. Listen to your breathing and keep it rhythmic. Make sure your arms, neck, and shoulders stay loose and relaxed. Tell yourself, "Only five minutes to go. It'll be over in no time."

# Tapering

Some people run for no reason other than the health and stress-reduction benefits they get from a regular training program. Other runners, of course, train to race. They construct elaborate training programs intended to get them ready for a season of competitive races—in track, cross-country, or on the roads. Or, perhaps, for a single big event like a marathon.

Either way, they use their training as a springboard to a peak effort. But peak efforts don't come easily. And they won't occur at all unless you follow a period of decreased training called tapering before your big race.

To understand why and how tapering is so important, think about the two primary things that happen when you do a training session. First, you lay the foundation for future improvements in your fitness level; this is called the training effect. The second thing that happens is more immediate and not so good, however: Your muscles and entire body get fatigued from the training. You could call this the fatigue effect.

The goal of all training is to organize your program so that the training effect stays ahead of the fatigue effect. One way to do this is through hard-easy training. Another way to do this, particularly before a big race, is through tapering. When you taper for a race, you're simply allowing the training effect from all your workouts to sprint far ahead of the fatigue effect.

You can taper by decreasing your mileage or decreasing your intensity. The former is more important than the latter. Indeed, research experiments have shown that you should continue to do small amounts of intense training—speedwork and tempo training—as you taper. This will guarantee that your legs don't forget how to run fast.

You'll gain the most by making significant reductions in your daily training. Two weeks before a marathon, for example, you should reduce your mileage by 50 percent and then by 50 percent again in the week before the race. If you started at 40 miles a week, cut back to 20 with one week to go and then to 10 miles in the week preceding the marathon.

Some runners find it difficult to taper, mostly for psychological reasons. They fear they'll get out of shape or gain weight if they cut back on their normal training. Not so.

In fact, there's a tried-and-true principle to reassure these people. There are no workouts you can do in the last two weeks before a race that will improve your race performance. But there are lots of workouts that will hurt your race. In other words, there's very little upside to the training you do in the final days and a very steep downside.

As in many other areas of running, it's always better to err on the side of caution.

## ❖ Principles ❖

1. You can't run a great race without tapering. Track and cross-country runners may require as little as a 3- to 4-day taper, but marathoners will need anything from 15 to 20 days.
2. When tapering, concentrate on cutting back your mileage. The less you run, the more your body will recover from previous training sessions and the better prepared it will be for a peak racing effort.
3. While decreasing your mileage, continue to do short but fairly intense training sessions at the pace (or slightly faster than the pace) you hope to maintain in your big race. These workouts will keep your legs from going flat.
4. Keep a positive attitude. Visualize the success you're going to have in your upcoming race. This is a time for your body to rest while your mind is shifting into high gear.
5. There's little you can do in the several days before a big race to improve your performance, so don't overtrain.

# The Start

After you've spent months getting ready for a race, you don't want to let any small last-minute mistakes ruin your preparations. To avoid such problems, you need to make sure you do everything right in the final hours, on the start line, and at the beginning of the race. The time to start concentrating is the night before.

Lay out and pack everything you'll need. As silly as it sounds, be sure you have your shoes, socks, racing shorts, and singlet. If your number has been mailed to you, pin it on the front of your singlet now. Other essentials include petroleum jelly, a towel, dry clothes, sunscreen, sunglasses, sports drink, and energy bars.

The night before is also the best time to make your plans for getting to the start location on time. Reread the entry blank, note the exact address of the registration area, and double-check the start time. Make your travel plans with an eye to arriving at the registration location at least an hour before the race start time. Set your alarm clock, and get going exactly as planned when you wake up the next morning.

After arriving at the race location, take care of any required registration, and then look for the bathroom. If you're like most runners, you'll have to visit the bathroom before the race. The sooner you go, the better. You don't want a last-second panic.

Start your warmup about 20 to 30 minutes before you go to the start line, but don't overdo it. Staying relaxed is the key. Go to the start line in the area posted for runners of your pace. On the start line, continue jogging in place and stretching lightly just to make sure you don't tighten up.

When you hear the start signal, begin repeating a simple mantra to yourself: "Stay focused. Stay relaxed." Go with the flow of the crowd around you. The initial goal is to avoid being tripped and to avoid tripping someone else. To do this, run in a straight line. Do not zigzag; this causes problems for you and others.

If it's a big race and the pack unfolds slowly, don't panic. It won't help to push through or around the runners in front of you. Eventually, you should be running free, and this is where your race really begins. Settle into a comfortable pace. Check your breathing. Try to make sure you're not running too fast, an almost universal problem at the beginning of races when the crowds and the adrenaline get you pumped up.

If you've lost several minutes at the start, don't try to make up the time. Doing that usually produces the opposite effect: You run too fast in the first half of the race and too slow in the second half. Instead, try to run at the pace that works best for you. Don't worry about anyone else; run your own best race.

## ❖ Principles ❖

1. Pack your gear bag, including shoes, clothes, and race number the night before the race. Double-check the race start time and location, and make appropriate travel plans for the next morning. Set an alarm clock.
2. Get your trip to the race started on time the next morning. Eat a light, easily digestible carbohydrate food an hour or two before the race. Take along some water or sports drink and some simple carbohydrate foods such as energy bars or bagels. Plan to arrive an hour before the race starts.
3. Once you're at the race location, complete any registration process and begin thinking about your bathroom needs. The sooner you can take care of this, the better you'll feel.
4. Line up at the appropriate pace sign for runners of your ability. While you wait for the start signal, stay relaxed but continue jogging in place and stretching lightly.
5. Don't panic if you can't run freely at the beginning of the race. Stay focused, stay calm, and, most important, stay on your feet. When the race opens up, don't get carried away and run too fast. Stick to your own best pace.

# Pace

In races longer than a mile, the best strategy is always to cover the distance at an even pace. Scientific studies consistently show that this is the best way to use available energy during the race. So we know that it works physically.

Even-pace racing also works psychologically. You should feel relatively comfortable for most of the race and even better as you pass other runners in the later stages.

The vast majority of runners, however, fail to run at an even pace. They go too fast at the beginning, and then, when they've depleted their energy, they slow down too much.

Learning to run at an even pace is a learning process. Few runners achieve it the first time. It's far more common to make the too-fast/too-slow mistake on a number of different occasions.

To break the habit, you only need three things. First, and most important, the belief that you can. Second, some training geared toward an even-pace race. And third, some practice in real race situations. Only practice makes perfect.

I can't supply the belief for you. I can only repeat what I said at the beginning of this chapter: Scientific research has consistently shown that even-pace racing produces the best results.

I *can* give you a good tough workout to help you learn even pace. Run three one-mile repeats. During the first one, concentrate on running at about your 5-K race pace or slightly slower. Take a five-minute jog rest between all of the repeats.

Do the same for the second and third repeats. During the third, you may find yourself struggling, perhaps losing form. If so, you probably ran the first repeat too fast. Make a mental note of this, and the next time you do the workout, run even more relaxed during the first repeat.

Now, take the workout to the race. At the start, stay totally calm and relaxed. The first half-mile is the most important. Run at the slowest pace that doesn't seem outright silly and uncomfortable.

As you fall into a nice rhythm, try to recapture the feel of that first, controlled mile in the workouts you've been running. (I'm assuming here that you're racing a 5-K; in a longer race, the first mile would be much more relaxed.) Monitor your breathing. It should remain smooth, consistent, regular. No gasping.

Keep the same pace in the second mile, even as things get tougher. Recall your workouts, where you stayed strong and controlled. In the third mile, you'll start catching a lot of runners who started too fast. Congratulations. The plan is working.

Don't sprint past these runners in a showy fashion; that would waste energy. Just motor along like a car on autopilot. When you pass one runner, focus your attention on catching the next one. Enjoy it. This is the way racing should be.

## ❖ Principles ❖

1. The best, most efficient way to run a distance race—both physically and psychologically—is at an even pace. Unfortunately, many runners never master this technique.
2. To achieve the ability to race at an even pace takes belief, training, and practice. The belief is often the hardest part, as many runners have started fast and finished slow so many times that they can't imagine a different way to race.
3. The best workout to learn even-pace racing involves mile repeats. Do three of them at about 5-K race pace. Concentrate on staying relaxed, strong, and controlled. Take a five-minute jog rest between repeats.
4. In your next race, focus first on staying completely calm at the start. If you don't get carried away in the first half-mile, you're making major strides already.
5. The rest of the way, try to recapture the feeling of those mile-repeat workouts. Don't race against anyone around you. Run within yourself at a hard but sustainable pace.

# Part XI

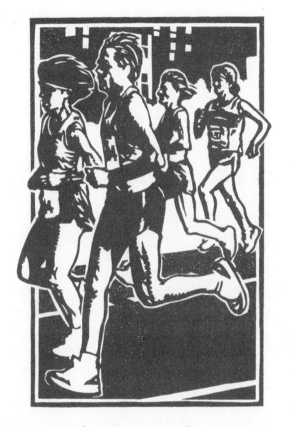

# The Marathon

# Commitment

The marathon is both the greatest challenge and greatest motivator in running. Everyone has heard of the marathon, most everyone has seen some of the world's best runners on TV in the Olympics or other races, and nearly everyone has heard that Oprah Winfrey and Al Gore have completed marathons.

As a result, the marathon is like a Mount Everest for average people. It's the pinnacle distance for runners but one that's accessible to almost anyone who laces up his training shoes on a regular basis.

Hundreds of thousands of runners enter their first marathons every year. Some are young, strong, and eager. Some are middle-age, confused about the meaning of life, and looking for events with which they can redefine themselves. Some are older but determined to maintain their vigor and endurance.

All yearn to tackle something heroic. Something they have an honest chance of achieving. But something that won't come easily. The marathon attracts people, says Jeff Galloway, a great marathon coach and former Olympian, "because it scares them." In other words, if you don't make the commitment and do the work, you won't finish the distance.

In marathon training, the commitment is the most important thing. Without it, you can't succeed, period. With it and a reasonable amount of luck and some steady training, you will succeed. The vast majority of marathoners, including first-timers, do complete the distance (as high as 95 percent, if the conditions are good).

The ones who lack commitment don't treat the marathon with enough respect. They might think, "Hey, if Oprah did it, how tough can it be?" They spend more time looking for shortcuts than taking their long runs. This will not work.

If you're a relatively inexperienced runner who hasn't been training very much, you may need as long as six months to get ready for your marathon. If you have more experience and more miles in the bank, you may need only eight weeks.

If your main goal is to finish the marathon in good physical shape, you'll only need to run two or three times a week. If you're aiming for something higher, such as a Boston Marathon qualifying time, you'll have to work out five or six times a week.

The point is, there's a training program that will work for you. The program itself isn't overly important. I've seen hundreds of them, and the ones from reputable sources are all quite good.

As far as I'm concerned, there are only two golden rules for marathon training. First, you must have a program that makes sense for you and takes into account your prior running experience and goals. Second, you must stick to the program. If you have the discipline and determination to stick it out, the training plan will lead you to the marathon success you're hoping for.

# ❖ Principles ❖

1. The marathon is both an Olympic event and an Everyman (and woman) event. Oprah did it and so can you, once you decide to make the commitment.
2. There are no secrets to marathon preparation. You need only two things: a plan and the commitment to stick to it. The plan isn't overly important; there are many good ones. The key is your own discipline and determination.
3. Depending on your prior fitness, you'll need as long as six months or as little as 8 weeks to get ready for a marathon. The vast majority of runners need 12 to 16 weeks to get ready.
4. Depending on your goal—that is, your hoped-for finish time— you'll have to run as little as two or three times a week or as much as five or six times a week.
5. Whatever goal you select, you'll encounter moments of fear and uncertainty. This is completely normal. Things will get better, and the thrill of finishing will erase any bad memories.

# Building Up

Training for a marathon is a case study in gradual adaptation to stress. You'll no doubt be running more than you ever have before—or, if you're a veteran marathoner, more than recently. At some point in your program, the primary thing you'll recognize is increased fatigue. You'll surely doubt your ability to ever cover 26 miles.

If you persist, however, you'll begin to feel your endurance growing. You'll come to understand, as you never have before, that training works by first making you weaker, then making you stronger and stronger.

To guarantee success, be sure to observe the 10-percent rule (for more information, see page 20). Keep in mind that your progress will add up quickly. After just eight weeks, your weekly mileage will more than double.

All marathon training programs put a special emphasis on long runs. Since the marathon represents a 26-mile challenge, it's no surprise that long runs will take center stage in your training program. If you run into obstacles in your program, such as illnesses or problems at work or home, you can salvage a marathon training program by completing the long runs even if you can't complete the other workouts.

Speedwork should be of little concern to marathoners. It's difficult to build both endurance and speed at the same time, and the former is challenging enough. To their surprise, many marathoners get faster anyway, because of their increased fitness (from additional training) and possible weight loss. (Don't lose too much weight, or you could sacrifice some of the strength and endurance you've been building.)

With the increased effort of the extra miles, you can't take a lot of other stress while training for a marathon. This isn't a good time for extensive travel, changing jobs, moving your family, building a garage addition, and so on. Concentrate on the big challenge you've accepted, and try to simplify the other areas of your life. It should go without saying that you need to pay extra attention to your sleep and nutrition while marathon training.

Similarly, I don't believe that runners should attempt to add new dimension to their fitness plans while training for a marathon. In other words, this isn't the best time to add weight training, bicycling, or swimming to workout plans. Save these for next year or your postmarathon recovery period. During the weeks and months of your training program, you'll have your hands full with the increased running workouts.

Don't forget that you need time to taper before race day. Most experts recommend that your training mileage should reach a peak three weeks before the marathon and should then decrease a substantial amount to help you build strength for the big day.

# ❖ Principles ❖

1. Marathon training involves a gradual adaptation to stress. Be sure to increase your mileage by no more than 10 percent per week.
2. All runners hit physical and psychological low points at some time in their training. Ride it out and stay confident. Things will get better, and you will go the distance.
3. Concentrate on your long run. In terms of preparing you for the marathon, this single workout represents about 80 percent of your training program. Don't worry about your speed. Just build your endurance.
4. Don't add other new wrinkles, like cross-training, to your program while getting ready for a marathon. Concentrate on the main event. Simplify your life, and pay special attention to your sleep and nutrition.
5. Begin your taper three weeks before race day. Remember, the taper is the most important part of your program. Even though you're doing less training, this is the time when your body gets strongest. Don't downplay the taper. It's crucial.

# Essential Element

The long run rests at the heart of every marathon training program. You haven't really started down the road to the marathon until you commit to a series of ever-longer runs. Once you have started, however, the road can take you as far as you want to go.

Every prospective marathoner has the same three questions about long runs. How far should I run? How often? How fast? You'll encounter other related questions along the way—Should I eat and drink? What should I do the next day?—but if you get the first three right, you'll accomplish about 98 percent of what you need to do on your long runs.

**Length.** Your first long run should be about 50 percent longer than your average midweek run. If your average run is four miles, then your first long run is a six-miler. Take it slow and easy, with walking breaks if necessary, and just aim to complete the distance.

Do your next long run a week later by adding an additional mile. Keep adding a mile a week until you reach 12 miles. After that, do long runs every other week, adding 2 miles a week. After completing a 20-mile long run, give yourself three weeks to taper for your marathon.

Many runners wonder how they'll ever finish a marathon if they haven't run 26 miles in practice. The answer is race-day magic. What this means, basically, is that you're capable of running both farther and more easily on your race day than on your training days. So, stay calm, be confident, and consider this: Doing extra-long training runs (beyond 20 miles) is more likely to injure you than to improve your endurance.

**Frequency.** The time off between long runs becomes more important as the long runs reach distances in the mid-teens. To fully recover from some inevitable aches and pains, and to build your reserves for your next long run, a gap of two weeks works much better than just one.

***Pace.*** Most runners should run their long workouts at the easiest, smoothest pace that feels comfortable. Don't run so slowly that your stride feels forced and awkward, but otherwise you shouldn't worry about going too slowly. It's much worse to go too fast, which could force you to abandon the workout or get injured.

The marathon world is full of formulas to help you determine your best long-run pace, but none of them are as important as your own internal comfort level. If the pace feels right and if you complete the distance with some energy, you're running the right pace.

The formulas do serve one purpose. They can help prevent you from going too fast. Here's one: Run your marathon-training long runs at a pace at least 1½ to 2 minutes per mile slower than your 10-K race pace. Follow this, and you should do fine.

## ❖ Principles ❖

1. Long runs are the essential element of marathon training. If you're not following a schedule of progressively longer long runs, you're not training for the marathon.
2. Your first long run should be 50 percent longer than your average midweek run, assuming this average run is in the 3- to 6-mile range. Your first long run should never be more than 10 miles.
3. Do your follow-up long runs once a week, adding 1 mile per week to the distance of the workout. Once you reach 12 miles, do your long runs every other week, adding 2 miles per week. Stop doing long runs when you reach 20 miles.
4. Don't worry about your pace on these long runs. Just stay as comfortable as you can. The whole idea is to run long and slow, not long and fast. A good guideline: Run 1½ to 2 minutes slower per mile than your 10-K race pace.
5. Give yourself at least a three-week taper after your longest run and before the marathon. Don't worry about the fact that you'll have to go six miles farther than you've ever run before. Race-day magic will help you reach the finish line.

# Yasso 800s

Most of the information I've passed along in this book came to me after years of trial and error. I heard about a particular workout or some other tip, used it myself, evaluated the results, tried it again with a slight variation. Eventually, I concluded that the idea had some merit . . . or it didn't.

I learned about Yasso 800s in a completely different manner. My co-worker Bart Yasso and I had traveled together to the Portland Marathon, where we were manning the *Runner's World* expo booth. At one point, when I showed up to relieve Bart, he said, "I have to go run my 800s to get ready for the Twin Cities Marathon."

Intrigued that Bart was running 800s to get ready for a marathon, I began to question him about the workout. It turned out that he was doing a type of marathon workout I had never before heard about. Not only that, but it had some unique numerical and physiological properties.

Basically, Yasso 800s are advanced marathon workouts that can help you predict your marathon condition or prepare for a specific goal. In other words, they can help you decide if you're ready to run three hours, four hours, five hours, or whatever your goal time is. Most marathoners have a goal time in mind, and I know of no other workout that can predict marathon readiness in this way.

Best of all, Yasso 800s are incredibly simple. The ultimate aim is to run 10 repeats of 800 meters, each in the same time as your marathon goal. Sort of. Here are two quick examples to help you see the connection. If you want to run a 3 hour and 10 minute marathon, you run your 800s in 3 minutes and 10 seconds; if you want to run a 4 hour and 30 minute marathon, you run your 800s in 4 minutes and 30 seconds. That's all there is to it.

Of course, you don't simply begin with 10 Yasso 800s. You work up to that number by first running 3 or 4 Yasso 800s and then adding 1 a week over six weeks. You do your last Yasso 800 workout—the one with 10 repeats—at least two weeks before your marathon. Between repeats, you walk or jog for approximately the same amount of time it takes you to run each 800.

Do this workout once a week and simply incorporate it into your normal marathon training. I usually do the Yasso 800s in the middle of the week, a long run on the weekend, and fill in the rest of my training as best I can. Don't forget to schedule in a day or two of rest each week.

A word of caution: Yasso 800s are great workouts, but they can't warp reality. They won't deliver you to your marathon goal if it's completely unrealistic. However, if you pick a tough but attainable goal, Yasso 800s will let you measure your progress toward that goal and will ultimately tell you whether or not to attempt it on race day. That's a tremendous contribution.

# ❖ Principles ❖

1. Yasso 800s are a unique form of tempo training that can help you achieve your marathon goal time. They can't produce miracles, however. Your goal time has to be realistic.
2. The ultimate aim of Yasso 800s is to run 10 repeats of 800 meters, each in the same time as your marathon goal time. It's just that the units change. You run 3 minutes and 20 seconds instead of 3 hours and 20 minutes, or 4 minutes and 30 seconds instead of 4 hours and 30 minutes.
3. Begin with three or four Yasso 800s at your goal time. Between repeats, walk or jog the same amount of time that it takes you to run the repeats. The workout should feel comfortable.
4. Each week, add one more 800, until you reach 10. The workout will become quite hard—but hopefully doable at this point.
5. If you can run 10 Yasso 800s at your marathon goal time, then go for that goal on race day. If you can't, make appropriate adjustments. You can always aim for a faster time in your next marathon.

# Taper

When runners decide to run a marathon, they expect it to be a serious challenge. The aches and pains. All the long runs. The constant concern about proper nutrition.

But you cope with these things because you know they're part of the deal. What most runners don't expect is the physical, and especially the mental, turmoil they're going to face in the last seven days before the marathon. In many ways, the tapering period is the toughest thing you'll go through.

Your training has been building and building, then it suddenly stops. But you don't get to run the race right away. Instead, you sit around anxiously awaiting a race that is over a week away.

You imagine that this should be a pretty nice thing after you've been training so hard for so long. After all, you deserve a little rest and relaxation. Instead, you start noticing pains that had escaped you previously; you can't sleep; you have no energy; and every three-mile jog serves no purpose other than to convince you that you'll never be able to complete the full marathon distance. How can three miles possibly be so difficult?

Before long, your taper begins to seem more like the week from hell than like the vacation you had been imagining. Congratulations. This is the final, sure sign that you're ready.

Experienced marathoners have learned that the taper week is something that they can and will survive. Eventually, it will be over and you'll get to run the marathon you've been thinking about for so long. Until then, the best and most important strategy is to stay calm and be confident.

If you've done the training, everything will come together on race day. Until then, you simply have to ride out the storm. You'll have days during taper week when you seriously question your sanity. You'll almost certainly think about dropping out of the marathon. You'll also consider taking sleeping pills (because you can't sleep), quitting your job (what's the point, you can't concentrate on anything), and making an emergency visit to the doctor to see what's wrong with you. And this is only the normal stuff that happens to all marathoners.

To keep yourself on track, simply do what you've been doing all along, but on a smaller scale. Run and exercise, but not very much. Continue eating lots of low-fat carbohydrates. Stay well-hydrated. Fill your spare time with favorite books, running videos, or the latest movies.

You'll have plenty of emotional ups and downs in the week before the marathon. But they'll all fade away like distant memories on race-day morning, when suddenly, magically, you'll start feeling great about 10 steps after the start.

# ❖ Principles ❖

1. The last week before a marathon—the taper week—seems as if it should be a joy, but most runners find it an emotional roller coaster. You'll survive it much better if you're prepared.
2. Don't be surprised if you notice aches and pains you haven't felt before, if you can barely finish a three-mile run, or if you feel incredibly fatigued and have trouble sleeping at night. These are all common during taper week. Don't worry; they magically disappear as soon as the marathon starts.
3. Reduce your running mileage to just two to four easy miles a day or every other day, depending on your schedule. On Wednesday or Thursday, do four two-minute repeats at your marathon goal pace.
4. Continue to eat lots of low-fat carbohydrates and to stay well-hydrated. Don't eat foods you're not accustomed to, which is one of the most common marathon mistakes.
5. Try to take your mind off the marathon with diversions like books, videos, movies, and so on. Do anything that you find fun and involving. Save your greatest mental focus for the race.

# Carbohydrate-Loading

Carbohydrate-loading originated in the labs of the military, not the sports world. Several Scandinavian countries grew tired of losing soldiers who couldn't make it through long exhaustive treks in deep snow. They commissioned their top scientists to improve the soldiers' endurance, and carbo-loading evolved as one of the best ways to acheive this.

Carbohydrate-loading works because it supercompensates the supply of readily available energy in the muscles. With this additional energy supply, soldiers can march farther and runners can run farther and faster.

In its original and most rigorous form, the carbo-loading routine called for three days of depletion followed by three days of supercompensation. Then you ran the marathon. Bingo!

The theory is that your muscles are more eager to soak up extra carbohydrates if they have first been starved for several days. This procedure works better in theory than in practice. As I mentioned in the previous chapter, the seven days before a marathon can be hellish. If you incorporate three days of carbohydrate depletion, things get even worse.

Instead, most marathoners have adopted the practice of carbo-loading for the last three days before the marathon, without carbo-depleting first. Nutrition and exercise studies show that this procedure can be just as effective as the full six-day deplete-load cycle. It's definitely the procedure I recommend.

Remember to eat basic, common carbohydrates that you're accustomed to. Don't get seduced by new, and perhaps heavily spiced, foods at ethnic restaurants in the city you're visiting. The same goes for the heavily promoted products and supplements at health food stores and marathon expos. Some of these are, in fact, great carbo and nutritional supplements, but the time to try them isn't on the eve of your race.

Fluids can be a good source of readily absorbed carbohydrates. You have to stay hydrated anyway, so you may as well pack in some extra carbos at the same time. Again, drink only those sports beverages you've used regularly in training. And if you mix your own drinks from a powder, resist the temptation to mix them stronger than recommended. If anything, slightly weaker would be better.

Last, most marathons begin early in the morning. If you don't eat something that morning, then you've failed to break the fast induced by your seven or eight hours in bed. You've let yourself get depleted instead of loaded.

I know you may have to set your alarm clock for an ungodly hour, but breakfast is important, so make time for it. Be sure to eat some simple low-fiber carbohydrates that are part of your everyday diet and won't bother your stomach. Toast, bagels, and oatmeal are some great examples.

## ❖ Principles ❖

1. Carbohydrate-loading can improve your endurance by giving your muscles an increased supply of readily available energy.
2. The early experimental version of carbo-loading recommended a three-day depletion phase followed by three days of supercompensation. In practice, this procedure can prove very difficult. Three days of carbo-loading can be just as effective.
3. Stick to carbohydrates you're accustomed to, even if your meals start to get repetitious and boring. Concentrate on old standbys like breads, bagels, pasta, rice, and potatoes.
4. Use commercially available sports drinks to keep yourself hydrated and carbo-loaded at the same time. If you prepare your own drink from a commercial mix, don't increase its strength, as this could create gastrointestinal problems.
5. Break the fast of your last night's sleep, or you risk starting the marathon depleted instead of loaded. Wake up early enough to have a light but satisfying breakfast.

# Final 24 Hours

The last 24 hours before the marathon are the most trying, needless to say. By this time, every moment of the day is consumed by thoughts of the race, and it seems difficult to do anything right. Walk around, and you fear that you're wasting energy you may need tomorrow. Lie down, and thoughts swirl through your head so quickly that you feel more exhausted than when walking about.

No wonder so many runners like the idea of following a step-by-step plan to make sure they get everything right. Here's an outline for your last 24 hours before a marathon that should get you to the start in ready-to-roll condition.

***Morning, race day minus one.*** Sleep as late as feels comfortable. Even if you don't sleep late, stay in bed and read. Eat a generous breakfast that's full of your favorite high-carbo foods like pancakes, oatmeal or other cereals, bagels, fruit, and juices.

Take a relaxing walk around town or explore the city where the marathon is being held. Carry a water bottle filled with sports drink, and sip from it regularly. Continue doing the same all day long.

***Afternoon, race day minus one.*** Get away and do something that diverts you, as long as it allows you to sit down, like watching a movie. Avoid museums; the slow walking and hard floors are deadly. Eat a light lunch and snack on carbohydrates whenever you feel the urge. Keep drinking from your water bottle.

No doubt, you'll want to visit the marathon expo at some time. In fact, you may need to pick up your number. Fine. But don't overstay your visit. Don't wander the expo halls endlessly. Have a nice look, then get back to your hotel room and get your legs up on a bed. Take a nap if you can. If you can't fall asleep, at least force yourself to lie on the bed and meditate (or breathe deeply and restfully) for 20 minutes.

***Evening, race day minus one.*** Attend the pasta party, visit a nice restaurant in town, or (most boring but smartest of all) order room service. After dinner, watch a movie in your room or go out to a nearby theater. Don't worry about going to bed early. You're not going to sleep well anyway, and the amount of sleep you get (or don't get) the night before a race has no effect on your performance. So just go to bed when you feel like it.

**Early morning, race day.** Make sure you do everything this morning with absolute clockwork precision. Count back from the hour when you have to be at the start (or perhaps on a bus to the start), and leave yourself plenty of time to get up, get dressed, have breakfast, fill a water bottle, make several bathroom visits, and get to the start (or the bus). You're going to be very nervous this morning. Don't compound things by starting late and rushing through everything. Get up early, stick to a schedule, follow an organized plan, and stay relaxed.

# ❖ Principles ❖

1. Carry a water bottle filled with sports drink with you the day before the race. Take sips from it regularly to make sure you keep yourself fully hydrated.
2. Eat three modest but carbohydrate-filled meals the day before the marathon. You shouldn't be stuffing yourself; simply stick to carbohydrate foods. Don't hesitate to carbo-snack in the midafternoon (eat cookies, for example) or to have a dessert at night.
3. Stay off your feet as much as possible the day before the race. Move around and get out of your room, but don't visit museums or do anything that puts you on your feet for hours at a time.
4. Visit the marathon expo to pick up your race number and feel the marathon energy, but don't overstay your visit. Expos can be crowded, hot, dry, and exhausting. You don't need this the day before the marathon.
5. Get up early enough on race-day morning to have a small but sufficient breakfast, make several bathroom visits, and get to the bus or starting line on time.

# Early and Middle Miles

Running a marathon is an exercise in energy management. The goal is to avoid all things hurried, wasteful, and exorbitant.

Begin the day right by getting to the start area reasonably early. Leave yourself plenty of time to use the bathroom, find a quiet place to rest, and locate your proper starting position. If it's chilly, bring throwaway clothing or a plastic garbage bag to keep you warm and dry until the start.

You don't need much warmup for a marathon since you'll be starting slowly. Just jog around for 10 or 15 minutes, stretch lightly, do your favorite calisthenics, and line up in your correct position behind the start.

Once the marathon gets underway, don't fight the pack. You could push your way forward or zigzag through the slowly moving throng, but it would be a colossal waste of effort. Relax.

At some point, you'll be able to run free—to run at your own pace—and this is where many marathoners make the classic mistake. You have so much pent-up energy and adrenaline that you lose all sense of pace. You run too fast. It feels effortless. You begin to make up some of the time you lost at the start. Hallelujah!

Sorry. This won't last for 26 miles. Slow down *now*. Running a few seconds too fast at the beginning of a marathon will cost you minutes later. Relax. Take your time. Enjoy the stroll. Check your pace at every mile marker, and adjust it the moment you notice you're going too fast.

If possible, run with a friend who has the same goal time as yours. Stick together and assign each other to be "pace police." If you notice a too-fast mile, slow down. Both of you.

Managing your energy in the early parts of a marathon also requires making stops every couple of miles for sports drinks. Studies have shown that the most important time to drink is early, not later when you're too dehydrated for it to make a difference.

Experts recommend that you consume six to eight ounces of water or sports drink every 15 to 20 minutes. I recommend sports drinks for the double payoff of water and carbohydrates.

If you need to jog or stop completely to drink a full cup, do it. Don't worry about the several seconds you lose. It's time well-spent.

You may or may not need extra fuel—gels, bars, hard candies—in the first 13 miles. Follow the practice you used in your most successful long runs. Be sure to wash down your gels and bars with water, not sports drinks (the combo would give you too much sugar at once, possibly causing stomach problems).

Always keep an eye on your watch, and stick to the plan. Run at a smooth, steady, comfortable pace. Divert yourself by looking around at the scenery. Enjoy the view.

## ❖ Principles ❖

1. Get to the start reasonably early. Don't arrive late, in a last-minute panic. Use the bathroom, and find a comfortable place to rest. Be sure to double- or triple-knot your shoelaces.
2. Begin your warmup 15 minutes before going to the start line. You don't need much—just enough to feel loose and relaxed. Find your correct start position.
3. When the marathon begins, go with the flow. Don't push and shove and zigzag your way forward. That would be a colossal waste of energy. Don't worry about the time you're losing. It's okay to subtract the minutes you lose in the early miles.
4. Once you can run free, zero in on your marathon goal pace. It may take you a couple of miles to hit it, but then stay steady. Check your watch at all mile markers, and slow down the moment you notice that you're running too fast. If you have to speed up to reach your goal time, run no faster than 10 seconds per mile below your mile pace.
5. Stop at aid stations every several miles for sports drinks. Slow to a walk to make sure you can drink six to eight ounces.

# The Wall

At some point, the marathon gets tough, but you knew that, didn't you? There wouldn't be much point in tackling the 26.2-mile distance if it didn't represent a significant challenge. And it certainly does, especially when you hit the wall.

Marathoners hit the wall at about the 20-mile mark. That's the point where your body exhausts the fuel supplies that have largely been stored in the muscles. To continue running smoothly past the 20-mile mark requires intense concentration and a good bit of smarts.

The best strategy is to diminish the wall as much as possible by running a steady, conservative pace in the early and middle miles. If you do this, you'll still have to fight through the fatigue of the last six miles, but it won't be nearly as bad as it is for those who start foolishly fast.

You may, for example, slow down 30 seconds per mile in the last six miles—not a big deal. It will only add 3 minutes to your total time for that distance. Whereas those runners who totally miscalculate their paces and therefore have to walk most of the last six miles will lose 30 to 40 minutes. Believe me, it happens all the time.

When you feel the wall-fatigue mounting, don't panic and don't fight it. Doing so will only make you feel worse, and you'll tighten up if you try to push harder. Instead, accept that you need to slow down a little. Often, a very slight change of pace is all it takes to make you feel much better.

Think positive. You've finished four-fifths of the distance, and you're not going to let anything stop you now. All you have to do is keep moving. It won't be long before the finish line gloriously appears in view.

You have to keep consuming sports drinks alone, or water with bars and gels. Carbohydrates are essential now. They go straight to your brain, which helps keep you alert, aware, and working on your strategy. Many marathoners find that sucking on glucose tablets or hard candies keeps them going through the last six miles, even though the actual amount of sugar they supply is small.

Your mind is your greatest ally at this point. Use it to remind your legs that there's only one mile to go—from mile 20 to mile 21, that is. Then one more from 21 to 22, and so on. By breaking the race down into small chunks at this point, you make everything so much easier.

Some runners like to recall favorite or typical training courses back home. The last six miles is basically just a run "to the river and back," or whatever works for you. Looked at this way, the last six miles amount to nothing more than an everyday jaunt.

Besides, Oprah Winfrey ran the marathon, and Vice President Gore finished one, too. If they did it, so can you.

## ❖ Principles ❖

1. The best way, by far, to beat the wall is to run a smart, steady pace—one that's realistic for your training and talent. Go out too fast in the early or middle miles, and you invite disaster.
2. Don't panic when you feel the first heavy wave of fatigue wash over you. Stay relaxed and calm, and let yourself slow down a little. Don't fight the fatigue. You can't win that battle. But run smart, and you can finish the marathon.
3. Continue drinking fluids and eating bars and gels. A glucose tablet or hard candy can provide a quick boost to your brain as well as to your legs.
4. Think positive at all times, and keep moving. Many runners experience a bad patch near the wall and are surprised to find themselves feeling better a mile or two later. Don't quit. Things can and will get better.
5. Put your brain in control. It's your best weapon at this point. Break the remaining miles into small chunks, and think about how often you have run a favorite six-mile course at home.

# Recovery

You cross under the finish-line banner at the end of the marathon, you can stop running at last, and someone places a finisher's medal around your neck. Your first thought is, "Thank goodness I don't have to run another step."

Your second thought should be about recovering from the marathon. Now is the time to begin that recovery process. The sooner you do, the sooner and more completely your body will bounce back from the incredible feat it has just accomplished.

To begin the process, continue doing exactly what you were supposed to do during the last three to six hours: drinking and eating. No matter how thoroughly you've attended to this during the marathon, you will have gotten dehydrated and depleted. Now is the time to replenish.

As earlier, your best choices are a sports drink (for water and carbohydrates) and carbohydrate foods (to replenish the energy in your legs). When you get the chance, but within an hour or two of finishing the marathon, it's also a good idea to eat some protein, such as low-fat yogurt, low-fat chocolate milk, or a tuna sandwich.

With the refueling under way, it's time to think about your legs. If possible, begin icing your calf muscles, knees, quadriceps, or other areas where you notice soreness and stiffness. You've seen video clips of baseball pitchers icing their elbows and shoulders immediately after a game, and you should do the same for your legs.

You might feel tempted to take a bath and celebrate with alcohol, but resist. The bath will increase your leg stiffness by promoting swelling around your muscles, and beer is a diuretic, not a rehydrating beverage.

In the days following the marathon, you'll wonder when to return to your running. The answer? When your body tells you to. But err on the side of caution.

Many marathon experts recommend that, rather than run in the days after the marathon, you should walk, do water exercises, or bicycle. I agree. Do something that gets you moving but doesn't pound your legs.

Let your leg comfort or discomfort guide you. You may barely be able to walk for several days after the race. You may feel more soreness two days after the marathon than the day after because of delayed-onset muscle soreness. This is normal.

After five to seven days, you should be able to return to running with relative comfort. But take it very easy. Even if you had a successful marathon and are eager to begin training for your next one, don't. You should wait at least two weeks before inching back into a normal training routine, and up to four weeks before doing long runs, speedwork, or races.

## ❖ Principles ❖

1. Even after you cross the finish, your recovery plan demands that you continue doing what you did during the marathon: drinking and consuming carbohydrates. If possible, also consume a light protein food an hour or two after the race.
2. As soon as possible, begin icing the sore, tight places on your legs—probably the backs of your lower legs and fronts of your upper legs. If you want, take an over-the-counter painkiller and anti-inflammatory like ibuprofen or aspirin.
3. You might feel tempted to take a relaxing warm bath or to celebrate with alcohol. Try to resist. The warm bath will encourage more swelling of your sore muscles, and alcohol is a diuretic, not a rehydrating fluid.
4. Return to exercise when your body tells you it's okay. Don't force anything. Consider non-weight-bearing activities like water exercising and bicycling before you begin running again.
5. After five to seven days, running should feel comfortable again. But don't resume your normal training for at least two weeks, and don't do speedwork, long runs, or races for a month.

Part XII

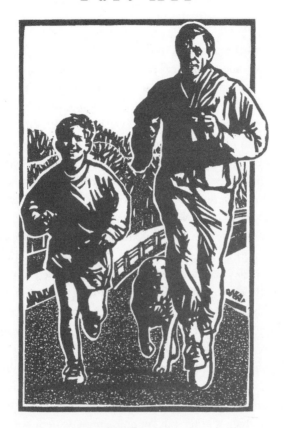

# A Lifetime
of Running

# Slowing Down, Feeling Great

Most of the chapters in this book have been about running farther, faster, and stronger. That's the sexy side of running, and it's what most people want to do at some point in their running careers. But running fast, at least in the relative sense, is easy when you're in your twenties and thirties. It's more difficult, and much more important, to learn to run slowly for the rest of your life.

In general, you have about seven years from the beginning of your running career to the time when you will run your fastest. That is, you can continue to improve for as long as seven years. And while you're improving, it's easy to stay motivated.

But everyone slows down eventually. Scientists haven't learned to stop the aging process—though running definitely helps—and the day comes when we all begin to lose muscle mass, key hormones, and other regulators that contribute to maximum performance. When this happens, you have a simple choice: Give up running because you're getting slower, or continue because you'll need it more than ever as you age.

It's obvious which choice I think you should make. In my own life (I'm 52 as I write this sentence), I find that in some ways I'm training harder now than I ever have. I'm not training faster, and I'm certainly not racing faster, but I'm doing more varieties of total-body training as I try to maintain as much strength and fitness as possible.

I believe that as we age, the psychological component of our health and fitness routines becomes much more important. Since we can't train with the thought that it will make us faster, we must find other motivations. I certainly run for the health benefits. I also run for reasons of vanity and sanity. I enjoy the occasional comments like "Gee, you don't look like you're 50." And I find that, in the middle of a hectic day of meetings and other commitments, my relaxed workouts provide much needed time-outs.

Let me add quickly that I still believe in high goals and challenges. I may be slower, but I still run marathons, and I'm still looking to do things I've never done before. The minute we stop challenging ourselves, we may as well stop living.

Each of us finds different reasons and challenges for running, and I'm not about to tell you what yours should be. But I will suggest that you think long and hard about them. Our motivations for running are absolutely central, because the physical act of running is much easier than the psychological energy it takes to do it.

As a result, we should plan our motivational strategy as thoroughly as we plot out a marathon training program. Take the motivation out of your running, and there is no running.

# ❖ Principles ❖

1. No one keeps improving forever. The most important years of your running career—or rather the decades, I hope— should be the ones that you spend getting slower and slower. Because these are the years when you will gain the most from the health and fitness benefits of running.
2. Your body will tell you when it's time to slow down, and there's no point in fighting it endlessly. Instead, adapt. Introduce new routines, seek new challenges.
3. Cross-training, recovery days, and strength training become much more important as you age. Use them all. In particular, find a twice-a-week strength-training routine that works for you. You simply want to retain as much muscle tissue as possible.
4. Continue to set exciting goals. Broaden your horizons. Don't try to run a personal best in the marathon, but run marathons in exotic locales. Find more friends who share your fitness goals.
5. Think every day about your motivational strategies. They're the key to your continued success. Read books that motivate you, collect quotes, adopt role models, and reward yourself regularly.

# Use It or Lose It

Life is about choosing. We can't influence everything we may like to, but we still face an endless array of decisions. And living with an aging body certainly presents its share of tough ones.

In the end, though, the biggest choice is a simple one: Do we give up or do we fight? Do we acknowledge that we reached our physical peak in our mid-twenties and that it's all downhill from there? Or do we fight for all the fitness and vitality that we can muster at every age?

Of course, no one can deny the biological process. You can't live forever. Some diseases seem horribly random, and others appear to have a strong genetic influence. Doing something, though, is far better than doing nothing at all. A positive, proactive attitude is the most important health attribute you can have. I'd take it over a good cholesterol ratio any day.

Too many runners give up on their training when they reach an age where they start slowing down noticeably. The stopwatch is a cruel master, and it can rob you of your motivation. But this is precisely the time when, because of the illnesses associated with aging, you most need to maintain a high level of fitness. Here's why (all these reasons are taken directly from a medical journal that is resting on my desk right now).

Exercise lowers the risk of depression, heart disease, high blood pressure, diabetes, osteoporosis, and some cancers.

Exercise controls obesity, a major risk factor for all of the above (and many other) diseases.

Exercise improves endurance, strength, flexibility, and joint range of motion in people with arthritis.

I'd like to add two more points to this already impressive list. First, exercise simply makes you feel better and more alive every day. Second, exercise gives you more energy.

Because this second point is counterintuitive, many people

simply refuse to believe it. They reason that 30 to 60 minutes of exercise a day has to make you more tired. They visualize runners collapsing at the end of a marathon. "So where's all this energy?" they ask sarcastically. Ha, ha. Very funny. But the fact remains that physical fitness improves energy levels all day, every day.

Last, a simple point about running. All of the above medical benefits accrue to those who exercise. You don't have to run. It's just that running, or a mixture of running and walking, is the quickest, easiest, most effective, and most all-weather method of vigorous exercise. When your goal is lifelong health and fitness, it pays to keep things simple and effective.

## ❖ Principles ❖

1. The most important thing you'll ever do with your running is to continue running . . . for the rest of your life. You'll run slower during these years, maybe even mixing together running and walking, but you'll also gain more physical and emotional benefits than ever before.
2. The list of medical benefits that exercise provides is almost endless, and running is the best lifelong exercise simply because it's the simplest, most time-efficient, and most effective.
3. Naturally, you'll have to adapt your training as you age. You should think less about performance and more about maintenance and injury prevention. When you feel the need for a rest day or a recovery day, take it.
4. You might switch to running every other day or every third day. You should definitely do more strength training, more cross-training, and more flexibility exercises.
5. By all means, keep running at the pace and level that seem appropriate to you. The energy you derive from your fitness program will spill over into other areas of your life, allowing you to stay active and involved in all the activities that are most important to you.